The Marriage Bargain: Women and Dowries in European History

The *Women & History* series:

- *Beautiful Merchandise: Prostitution in China 1860-1936,* by Sue Gronewold

- *The Empire of the Mother: American Writing about Domesticity 1830-1860,* by Mary P. Ryan

- *Women, Family, and Community in Colonial America: Two Perspectives,* by Alison Duncan Hirsch and Linda Speth, with an Introduction by Carol Berkin

- *Votes and More for Women: Suffrage and After in Connecticut,* by Carole Nichols, with a Foreword by Lois Banner

- *A New Song: Celibate Women in the First Three Christian Centuries,* by JoAnn McNamara

- Dames Employées: *The Feminization of Postal Work in Nineteenth-Century France,* by Susan Bachrach

- *Women and the Enlightenment,* by Margaret Hunt, Margaret Jacob, Phyllis Mack, and Ruth Perry, with a Foreword by Ruth Graham

- *The Marriage Bargain: Women and Dowries in European History,* edited by Marion A. Kaplan

The Marriage Bargain: Women and Dowries in European History

Marion A. Kaplan
Editor

Copublished by
The Institute for Research in History and The Haworth Press, Inc.

The Marriage Bargain: Women and Dowries in European History has also been published as *Women & History*, Number 10, 1985.

Library of Congress Cataloging in Publication Data
Main entry under title:

The Marriage bargain.

Published also as no. 10 of Women & history.
Includes bibliographical references and index.
Contents: From brideprice to dowry in Mediterranean Europe / Diane Owen Hughes—Women, dowries, and capital investment in thirteenth-century Siena / Eleanor S. Riemer—Trousseau as treasure / Jane Schneider—[etc.]
1. Dowry—Europe—History—Addresses, essays, lectures. 2. Bride price—Europe—History—Addresses, essays, lectures. 3. Marriage—Europe—History—Addresses, essays, lectures. 4. Women—Europe—Economic conditions—Addresses, essays, lectures. 5. Women—Europe—Social conditions—Addresses, essays, lectures. I. Kaplan, Marion A.
HQ1017.M37 1984 392′.5′094 84-15707
ISBN 0-86656-311-3

To Ruth

Who has endowed my life with love and happiness

The Marriage Bargain: Women and Dowries in European History

Women & History
Number 10

CONTENTS

Acknowledgement

I feel extremely fortunate to be part of a warm community of women scholars, colleagues, and friends, who have encouraged me with their moral support and their intelligent advice and insights. They have fostered my work in a demonstration of their own generosity as well as of women's traditional nurturing and caretaking roles, and I know that, in part, they have been able to do this because of the inspiration and strength they drew from the women's movement. In particular, I want to thank the members of the Institute for Research in History, especially the participants in the Institute's Women's History Research Group, and my friends, Renate Bridenthal, Deborah Hertz, Paula Hyman, and Alexandra Weinbaum. I am grateful as well to the editors of *Women & History,* Lois Fenichel, Alice Miller, and Eleanor Riemer, for their careful reading and editing of this volume. Finally, as always, I would like to thank Jay L. Kaplan for his painstaking readings of my essay and introduction as well as for his partnership in maintaining a home and family while I was preparing this volume. To Ruth, who has seen her mother at the typewriter for what must have seemed an interminable time to a five-year-old, my thanks for her patience, and my love for being "just the way you are."

Marion A. Kaplan

The Marriage Bargain: Women and Dowries in European History

Introduction

Marion A. Kaplan

"Love and marriage, love and marriage, go together like a horse and carriage. . . ," or, at least, sound more harmonious than "money and marriage." Americans, in particular, today regard love as the paramount element in the decision to marry, despite the persistent influence of class, ethnic, religious, and educational considerations. In fact, from a broad historical perspective, love has had a rather weak association with—and has very rarely preceded—marriage. At least until the age of the automobile, financial and social considerations were at the heart of the decision to marry.[1] Yet this point is easily lost when romantic love is daily glorified in the arts and popular entertainment and in the mating rituals of a society which, although plagued by high rates of divorce, clings tenaciously to the ideal of individual fulfillment through marriage. Even if the freedom to choose a mate is more circumscribed by social determinants than is admitted in popular mythology and even if the durability of love is tenuous, there is an apparently endless fascination with its permutations.[2]

In contrast, there is little popular interest in, or awareness of, the less glamorous but historically more lasting aspect of marriage—the dowry. Scholars, however, are increasingly aware of the dowry's significance. Numerous anthropologists have studied bridewealth and dowry, and historians of western societies have recently begun to investigate this essential side of the marriage bargain.

In Western societies, the dowry has been a payment made by the bride's family in cash, goods, or property to the groom. Once married, the wife generally had no access to her dowry, which was controlled by her husband for the duration of the marriage. But its size and the limited control she could exert might influence her status vis à vis her mate. In many instances, the dowry returned to the wife upon the husband's death, or, in fewer cases, desertion. Dowries were a means of contributing to the new household. They were also a way of transmitting wealth from parents to children, what has been called the bride's "pre-mortem inheritance."[3]

However, the dowry always signified much more than a transfer of funds: recent investigations of the dowry in various periods and places reveal its centrality to the history of Western women. The dowry was the most significant factor in a young woman's marriageability, and, hence, in affecting her future. Through the dowry, the political, economic, and social determinants which limited women's agency are revealed. Studies of the dowry address issues of women's status, their roles in the family, the family economy, and the economy at large. Such studies force us to ask questions about women's power and autonomy; women's relationships to parents, husbands, and children; and women's (and men's) marriage and fertility patterns. Further, studies of the dowry raise important issues of family history, from the foundation of the family economy to the reproduction of the family; from the power relations between genders and generations to the realm of affection among family members.[4] Also, these studies provide a material background against which the history of sexuality may be interpreted. Just as inheritance laws affected family formation and sexual patterns,[5] so, too, dowry customs, laws, and fluctuations may have reshaped individuals' intimate experiences. Finally, political and economic changes affected the history of the dowry, but dowries were also used to alter political constellations and to build economic alliances. Therefore, a focus on dowries can also provide social historians the tools with which to approach political and economic history.

The reasons for the neglect until recently of the history of the dowry help to illuminate its nature and significance. Historians have had difficulties finding sources, scattered among state, church, and private holdings, and, of course tracking verbal agreements concluded with a handshake is an impossibility. The dearth of research may also result from the fact that the nineteenth-century bourgeoisie, which praised romantic love and defended itself against socialist critiques of financially-arranged marriages, was unable to expose dowries to historical analysis, seeing them as mildly shameful.[6] The importance of dowries for the lives of women may have also had to await analysis by scholars of women's history or, perhaps, by women historians. Male historians of preceding generations, middle-class professionals and most likely the recipients of handsome dowries, may have been threatened by the topic of the influence of money on family life and intimate relationships. Finally, as Jane Lambiri-Dimaki suggests (see *essay five*), in societies where the dowry can still be investigated, the social sciences are in their formative stages, and where the social sciences are most developed, the dowry has almost entirely ceased to exist and must be painstakingly reconstructed.

The articles in this volume underline the enormous complexity of a topic which stands at the intersection of women's, family, and social history and they set forth provocative themes which merit further exploration and discussion. They span over a thousand years of Western history, focusing on the institution of the dowry among patricians and artisans in the Mediterranean cities of the eleventh and twelfth centuries (*Hughes, essay one*); the middle and upper classes in thirteenth-century Siena (*Riemer, essay two*); the Sicilian peasantry in the nineteenth century (*Schneider, essay three*); the Imperial German bourgeoisie (*Kaplan, essay four*); and Greek workers and farmers today (*Lambiri-Dimaki, essay five*). The articles illuminate the ways in which families protected their lineage and property, endeavoring to maintain or enhance their class status by matching a "promising" young man of appropriate status and good economic prospects with a financially well-endowed young woman. They underline the controls—particularly arranged marriages and the threat of disinheritance—that noble, bourgeois, and propertied peasant families exerted over daughters (and sons) to ensure the continuity of existing social relations. Also, they detail the broader economic and social structures within which young women married, and the degree to which the institution of the dowry structured courtship and marriage.[7]

These studies also suggest that dowries changed with the various stages of capitalism and varied in size with vacillations in the economy. Moreover, they raise the difficult and important question of what caused the rise, decline, or persistence of the dowry in different eras, regions, and among different classes of the population. Further, they point out how political conditions (the rise of the nation-state, warfare, the consolidation of political elites) caused fluctuations in the size and importance of the dowry. They also show how the exchange of dowries contributed to more cohesive political elites. Most strikingly, they describe a vast "traffic in women" as commodities, with economic, social, and, sometimes, political attributes.[8]

The dowry was known by the ancient Hebrews, although *bride-price* (*môhar*)—the groom's payment to the bride's family—was the legally required settlement.[9] Greek parents gave dowries with their daughters as did the Romans, until the Germanic invasions in the fifth century caused the Germanic brideprice to take precedence over the dowry for approximately five centuries. Yet, as early as the sixth century, in Burgundian, Visigothic, and Salic laws,[10] there was a gradual evolution from the brideprice to the *bridegift,* a marriage payment presented by the groom to the bride, rather than to her parents.[11] The bridegift provided for the economic security of women subsequently deprived of their husbands' support. Suzanne Wemple suggests that this improvement in women's economic rights was one of the most important developments in the history of Merovingian women. She argues that this evolution to bridegift was related to the growth of state power; Germanic leaders intended "to weaken the power of the kin by taking over the protection of the weak. . .in this case women who had been repudiated or had lost their husbands."[12]

In about the eleventh century, the burgeoning cities of the Mediterranean region abandoned the marriage customs imposed by the Germanic invaders in favor of the dowry. Diane Owen Hughes (*essay one*) explores the transition from brideprice to dowry by looking into the laws, charters, and social behavior of the patricians and artisans of the eleventh and twelfth centuries in Italy, southern France, and Catalonia. Hughes underlines the connections between commercial developments, a "crisis of status" (a fluid situation in which wealth and status were not balanced), and the need for economic and kin alliances. The dowry, she notes, played a key role in bestowing status and forging alliances. The size of the dowry indicated the bride's family's social and economic standing, and a large endowment could raise the status of the wife and her family. It is likely that a sizeable dowry insured the wife's family's involvement in her marriage, in order to protect her and their investment in the new household. Anthropologists have long identified gift giving—for example in marriage exchanges—as a means of exerting power.[13] This theme emerges strongly in Hughes' essay, as well as in the other articles. Finally, Hughes' evidence suggests that dowries were particularly crucial during a period of economic and social mobility, when those with new money sought status and those with status sought wealth either to maintain or regain their positions.

Like Hughes, Riemer (*essay two*) recognizes the correspondence between the commercial revival of the late middle ages in Italy and the return of the dowry. In her study of thirteenth-century Siena, she notes that this revival first brought increased legal and economic rights to middle- and upper-class women. She underscores male agency in the retrenchment of these rights, suggesting that laws limiting women's rights over their dowries were instituted by men who felt their economic and lineal interests threatened by women's control over property. Riemer also discusses the dowry as a "bridge between women's traditional status in the family and their roles in the new economy." The dowry, which was returned to a woman when her marriage ended, was women's "most regular and valuable source of capital for commercial ventures." Her essay highlights the relationship between women's power and autonomy and the extent to which they could exercise control over their dowries.

For historians of women, the studies by Hughes and Riemer are worth attention because they demonstrate how variations in women's status and power can be accounted for by particular economic and political factors. This can also be seen in research into dowries in medieval Ragusa (1235-1460).[14] There, in the midst of commercial growth, the elite reacted to a period of dowry inflation by using dowries to redistribute property broadly among wealthy families. Thus, it promoted further economic growth and forged cohesive economic and familial alliances. In this process, elite women received an increasingly larger share of their dowries in the form of jewels, ornaments, gold, and silver. This was not only a hedge against financial calamities, but more importantly, one which women controlled exclusively—an ultimately power-enhancing development for women. Similarly, in early Renaissance Venice (1300-1450) inflated dowries augmented the patrician wife's prestige and power.[15] Furthermore, Venetian state levies on private wealth forced fathers to seek financial help in assembling daughters' dowries, which in turn promoted closer kin relations, as fathers turned to relatives outside the direct male lineage for contributions. Thus, state policy affected the accumulation of dowries and the very identity of the donors. In Venice, an intricate web of political and economic conditions converged upon the dowry, shaping the social relationships among kin to increase "non-lineage ties of affection and interest."[16]

These examples, however, should not mislead us into thinking that the assertion of state or elite power necessarily improved women's position. In rural areas outside of Italy from the mid-twelfth to the mid-thirteenth century for example, the political order limited women's economic control. Feudal lords, intent on providing economic rights to their vassals, curtailed women's property rights, particularly over their dowries.[17]

Dowries were not only affected by political and economic developments, they, in turn, influenced broader social and demographic patterns.[18] In early modern France and England, for example, the need to save for the dowry resulted in later marriages among artisans and peasants. The dowry was a foundation of the family economy, and if peasant or artisan parents could not provide their daughters with dowries, the young women had to wait for their deaths to receive a settlements or had to work until they themselves accumulated enough money or goods.[19] Both alternatives seem to have raised the average age of marriage, while functioning as a kind of birth control as well. Among the propertyless, however, women generally worked before and during marriage.[20] Among these wage workers, the coming of domestic industry and the concomitant increase in jobs and cash wages as, for example, in seventeenth-century England, encouraged earlier marriages and more children.[21]

At least until World War I, saving for her dowry was an important aspect of a young working woman's life. In parts of Europe, a dowry was even required by law.[22] After the War, the expectation that a woman would continue to earn a wage during the early years of her marriage relaxed the need for her premarital saving. But the dowry was not abandoned entirely. The German peasantry continued the tradition of the dowry at least until World War II, with only the poorest unable to provide some sort of dowry or, at least, a trousseau.[23] The Sicilian peasantry, too, held to the dowry, which provided social status and separated the better-off from the "very poor." To this peasantry, embroidered trousseaux, which were objects of value with significant liquidity, functioned like dowries. They enhanced the social status of the bride and her kin and supported cultural codes of chastity and leisured womanhood by keeping women busy (and, therefore, "virtuous") but not employed, before marriage. Jane Schneider's essay (*essay three*) depicts the interrelationship between economic depression in late nineteenth-century Sicily, demographic transition, the lack of state or public social welfare institutions, and the intense devotion to embroidered trousseaux.

In France, the dowry was almost a universal institution, even among servants, laborers, and tenant farmers, until the interwar era.[24] Only the poorest urban industrial workers had no dowries, and, as a result, many of them did not marry at all. However, as some of them rose to the ranks of artisans, they, too, accumulated dowries and married. Consequently, marriage was seen by the bourgeoisie as a means of instilling love of property in the poor; a love which was nowhere more open and obvious than in the bourgeois marriages of the late nineteenth century. "For the great majority of the bourgeoisie, marriage is the greatest financial operation of their lives" wrote an observer of the French scene.[25] With the growth of industrial capitalism, the industrialists of the French Nord married off their children to their rivals, thus expanding family business and eliminating competition.[26]

During a period of depression and rapid capital accumulation in Imperial Germany, dowries took on added meaning for a successful and enterprising bourgeoisie eager to invest, as well as for a caste of nobles and higher civil servants whose fortunes had declined (Kaplan, *essay four*). Parents insured their family fortunes by arranging marriages, relenting only slowly to the pressures of "romantic love." Women's fate hung on the size of their dowries: the greater the sum, the "better" they married, and the greater their status vis-à-vis their husbands and in-laws. The corollary to this was also true: without an education or the means to support themselves, those with meager endowments entered less desirable marriages in weaker positions, chose propertyless marriages, or remained single, and often destitute, for life. For Germany's Jewish minority, and for ethnic and religious minorities in general, dowries served additional functions. Ethnic and religious groups often displayed distinct economic profiles (in the case of German Jews, preponderantly in commercial enterprises) and a commitment to endogamy. For the most part, dowries were used to maintain group cohesion, and class cohesion within the group, but this did not prevent the wealthiest from using a large dowry to marry out if they wished.

Only when women began to reenter the economy as paid workers on a large scale in advanced capitalist societies did the pursuit of dowries decline. Still, the dowry system is in evidence today in less industrialized areas of Europe. In analyzing the function and structure of the dowry as an institution in Greece, Jane Lambiri-Dimaki (*essay five*) shows that farmers as well as the working and lower middle classes continue to uphold the custom of dowry.[27] Only more privileged sectors of society accept the idea that a woman's education is her dowry. She finds that, ironically, the traditional institution of dowry encourages female emancipation: in order to accumulate a dowry, urban middle-class and rural peasant women must take jobs outside their homes, tasting independence for the first time.

Others have suggested that the dowry, particularly when it is linked with a "bride-built" house, given by the bride's relatives (as among Greek Cypriot villagers), reaffirms male dominance and the idea of motherhood as woman's destiny. The house enshrines the bride's roles as wife and mother, the perpetuator of the nuclear family which will reproduce the bourgeoisie with its patterns of private consumption, property ownership, and bourgeois values. At the same time, the woman's seclusion in the house secures male authority. Thus, class interests are furthered by a "residual" ideology of female subordination and male honor.[28]

* * *

To understand the complexity of the marriage gift, we have to view it in historical perspective, examining the continuities and discontinuities in this social institution from place to place, and from one era to another. What was the meaning of the dowry, for example, in different regions of Renaissance Italy and to different classes in these areas? What was its significance for individuals within a given class—to daughters, wives, husbands, parents—before and after the growth of the nation state or the rise of commercial, and then, industrial capitalism?

A sketch of the history of the dowry not only reveals the relationship of global forces such as the economy and the state, to the marriage gift, but the effect this gift had on social relations: the balance of power between wife and husband, parents and children, and among extended kin. As Jack Goody has pointed out,

> transmission. . .is not only the means by which the reproduction of the social system is carried out (insofar as that system is linked to property. . .); it is also the way in which interpersonal relations are structured.[29]

Further research must examine power relations within the family and the community in the context of gender and generation. Also, we must try to discover the relationship, if any, between the emotional bonds within the married couple and between generations—for example, what has been called the rise of "affective individualism," particularly after 1700[30]—and the form and function of dowries.

Finally, the marriage endowment reflects the position of women—their status, wealth, and autonomy—as daughters, wives, and mothers. What was the status of the daughter whose birth "fill[*ed*] a father's heart with fear"[31] because of the large dowry which her marriage would require? How were dowries, or the threat of their loss, used to constrain rebellious daughters? Whereas daughters might suffer from the demands of the marriage market, might not wives with generous endowments have wielded more power in their marriages? Similarly, was a woman's position enhanced when she could bequeath property to her children? Further, even wives who did not control their dowries could, in most instances, claim them in case of separation or divorce—could this have inhibited male whim and protected women?

Women's position was shaped by patriarchal society and ideology as well as by the nuclear family: it is within these contexts that the dowry must be examined. Further research is required into the terms of the relationship between the ideology of women's subservience and the dowry as a rational economic system for the social reproduction of wealth. Moreover, although property and power relations in a marriage pass through a number of stages, most existing studies take a static view. While it is historically true that wives, in general, could not assert their economic independence until their husbands died, there are significant exceptions (see, for example, *essays two* and *four*). Future research must include longitudinal studies of the property relations in marriages over the family lifecycle. Finally, the limitations of individual case studies point to the need for explicitly comparative analyses of the role of dowries among different classes in different eras and geographical locations. Hopefully the studies in this volume will shed light on the nature, quality, and social significance of the marriage bargain and will lead toward a feminist conceptual framework for approaching the history of the dowry.

REFERENCES

1. These are still the most important determinants in the United States, particularly for its upper class, whose cohesiveness is demonstrated by the high percentage of marriages within the Social Register.

2. See: William J. Goode, "The Theoretical Importance of Love," *American Sociolog-*

ical Review, 24, no. 1 (February 1959): 38-46. Goode discusses the structural patterns by which societies keep "love" in check.

3. Jack Goody and S.J. Tambiah, *Bridewealth and Dowry,* Cambridge Papers in Social Anthropology 7 (Cambridge, 1973).

4. H.J. Habakkuk notes that inheritance systems, of which dowries are a part, influenced family size and relations between members, as well as population mobility and productivity. See "Family Structure and Economic Change in Nineteenth-Century Europe," *The Journal of Economic History* 15, no. 1 (1955): 4-5.

5. Ellen Ross and Rayna Rapp, "Sex and Society: A Research Note from Social History and Anthropology," in *The Powers of Desire: The Politics of Sexuality,* eds. Ann Snitow, Christine Stansell, Sharon Thompson (New York, 1983), 57.

6. For an excellent analysis of the Owenite critique of marriage, see Barbara Taylor, *Eve and the New Jerusalem: Socialism and Feminism in the Nineteenth Century* (New York, 1983). See also, Friederich Engels, *The Origin of the Family, Private Property and the State* (1884; reprint, New York, 1972) and the introduction by Eleanor Leacock.

7. Indeed, dowries function to control courtship and marriage in parts of the world today. The most extreme examples of this, the recent phenomenon of bride burning or "dowry deaths" in India, occur because of the groom's family's dissatisfaction with the amount of dowry brought by the new bride. If the bride does not satisfy her in-laws' avarice, they conspire to kill her in the hope that their son will remarry and get a second, larger dowry. In New Delhi alone, reported cases of such deaths reaches an alarming 610 in 1982 (and many are not reported). *India Today,* October, 1983. See also, "Burn her and try again," *Economist,* July 14, 1979, p. 59.

8. Gayle Rubin, "The Traffic in Women: Notes on the 'Political Economy' of Sex, in *Toward an Anthropology of Women,* ed. Rayna R. Reiter (New York, 1973), 157-210.

9. For futher discussion of the dowry among Jews, see: S.D. Goitein, *A Mediterranean Society: the Jewish communities of the Arab world as portrayed in the documents of the Cairo Geniza,* vol. 3, *The Family* (Berkeley, 1978); Jacob Katz, "Family, Kinship, and Marriage among Ashkenazim in the Sixteenth to Eighteenth Centuries," *Jewish Journal of Sociology,* no. 1 (April, 1959): 4-22.

10. Suzanne Fonay Wemple, *Women in Frankish Society: Marriage and the Cloister, 500 to 900* (Philadelphia, 1981).

11. For the many variations of brideprice, bridewealth, and dowry, see Jack Goody, *The Development of the Family and Marriage in Europe* (Cambridge, 1983). He reminds us that one type of gift from the groom did not exclude the other kind (p. 206) and that payments *to* the father could also be an endowment of the bride (p. 242). See, in particular, Appendix 2, "From brideprice to dowry?"

12. Wemple, *Women in Frankish Society,* 44. See also, Viana Muller, "The Formation of the State and the Oppression of Women: Some Theoretical Considerations and a Case Study in England and Wales," *The Review of Radical Political Economics, URPE,* 9, no. 3 (Fall 1977): 7-21. Muller argues that the development of the state and the concomitant dissolution of corporate kin groups resulted in the development of private property, the nuclear family, and patriarchy. She suggests that during this process women lost autonomy and became dependent on their husbands. Fortunately, new customs and laws "softened the blow" (pp. 16-17).

13. Marcel Mauss, *The Gift: Forms and Functions of Exchange in Archaic Societies* (New York, 1967).

14. Susan Mosher Stuard, "Dowry Increase and Increments in Wealth in Medieval Ragusa (Dubrovnik)," *Journal of Economic History* 16, no. 4 (December 1981), 795-812.

15. Stanley Chojnacki, "Dowries and Kinsmen in Early Renaissance Venice," *Journal of Interdisciplinary History* 4 (Spring 1975): 571-600.

16. Ibid., 575.

17. David Herlihy, "The Medieval Marriage Market," in *The Social History of Italy and Western Europe, 700-1500,* ed. David Herlihy (London, 1978), 9.

18. J. Hajnal, "European Marriage Patterns in Perspective," in *Kinship,* ed. Jack Goody

(Middlesex, England, 1971), 140-47. David Herlihy has suggested that, in turn, social and demographic patterns may have influenced the size of dowries. See, "Medieval Marriage Market," p. 18 and Diane Owen Hughes' discussion of his theory in this volume.

19. Louise A. Tilly and Joan W. Scott, *Women, Work, and Family* (New York, 1978), 25, 34 (regarding the seventeenth century).

20. Ibid., 43.

21. Ibid., 25. The growth of commercial agriculture may have had the same effect in other areas.

22. Heilwig Schomerus, "The Family Life-Cycle: a Study of Factory Workers in Nineteenth-Century Württemberg," in *The German Family* ed. Richard J. Evans and W.R. Lee (London, 1981), 189.

23. Robert Lee, "Family and 'Modernisation': the Peasant Family and Social Change in Nineteenth-Century Bavaria," and Gerhard Wilke and Kurt Wagner, "Family and Household: Social Structures in a German Village between the Two World Wars," in Evans and Lee, *The German Family*. See also, David Sabean, "Aspects of kinship behaviour and property in rural Western Europe before 1800," in Jack Goody, Joan Thirsk and E.P. Thompson, eds., *Family and Inheritance: Rural Society in Western Europe, 1200-1800* (Cambridge, 1976), 96-111. Sabean suggests that as peasants became more involved in urban market transactions more funds were made available for cash endowments. Brides began to bring more into the marriage, matched equally by grooms. A "conjugal community" resulted in which brides acquired the right to inherit the farm.

24. Theodore Zeldin, *France 1848-1945, Ambition and Love* (Oxford, 1979), 18.

25. Paul Bureau, 1927, quoted by Zeldin, ibid., 291.

26. Ibid., 65. See also: Bonnie G. Smith, *Ladies of the Leisure Class: The Bourgeoises of Northern France in the Nineteenth Century* (Princeton, New Jersey, 1981), 57-63.

27. The government of socialist Prime Minister Andreas Papandreou has succeeded in revamping the Greek Family Code. For the first time, the requirement that women have dowries has been abolished.

28. Caroline Ifeka-Moller, "Changes in property transfer among Greek Cypriot villagers," in *Man* 11 (1976): 592-94. See also, Peter Loizos, "Changes in Property Transfer among Greek Cypriot Villagers," *Man* 10 (1975): 503-19.

29. Jack Goody, introduction to *Family and Inheritance,* 1.

30. Laurence Stone, *The Family, Sex and Marriage in England, 1500-1800* (New York, 1977). Women's legal rights over their dowries and possessions declined between the sixteenth and eighteenth centuries (see Natalie Zemon Davis, "Women on Top," in Natalie Zemon Davis, *Society and Culture in Early Modern France* (Stanford, 1975), 126.) recouping some thereafter. The relationship of their "rights" to affective interactions within the couple needs further research.

31. Dante, referring to fourteenth century Florence, as quoted by Diane Owen Hughes in this volume.

From Brideprice to Dowry in Mediterranean Europe

Diane Owen Hughes

> The dowry is brought by husband to wife, not by wife to husband. Parents and kinsmen attend and approve of the gifts, gifts not chosen to please a woman's whim or to deck a new bride, but oxen, horse with reins, shield, spear and sword. For such gifts [a German] gets his wife . . . Tacitus, *Germania,* 18.

I

In ancient times the Greco-Roman world, in its adherence to a system of dotal marriage, distinguished itself from the barbarians who hovered on its borders and who gave bridewealth for their wives, not dowry to their daughters. Aristotle—perhaps recalling Homeric accounts of marriages like that of Hector, who married Andromache out of the house of Eëtion "when he provided great bridewealth [*hedna*]"[1]—claimed that the Greeks had once "bought their brides from each other." And some have contended that after they gave up capturing them, so, too, did the early Romans.[2] As Lévi-Strauss has seen in bridewealth a mark of the transition to complex structures, so some scholars have pointed to dowry as a sign of the change from a tribal, migratory, heroic age to the familial, settled, classical period, a progress visible in the Homeric record itself. For them the *hedna* that Penelope might lose if she remarried before Odysseus' fate was known, which is described as what "fittingly follows a dear child," is, as its name suggests, all or part of her bridewealth, subsequently bestowed on her by her own kin in

"From Brideprice to Dowry in Mediterranean Europe," by Diane Owen Hughes is taken from the *Journal of Family History*, Fall 1978, Vol. 3, No. 3

the form of dowry; and it stands midway between the *hedna* with which heroes like Hector got their wives and the "seven well-peopled cities" with which Agamemnon promised to dower one of his daughters on her marriage to Achilles.[3]

Others would deny that Greco-Roman society knew brideprice.[4] Finley has persuasively argued for the Homeric period that *hedna* had no relation to a fixed or customary brideprice, but that it and dowry were complementary parts of an elaborate gift exchange, which solemnized and characterized—if it did not legitimize—Homeric marriage. Real transition came later, perhaps in the seventh or sixth centuries, in the shift from the "*oikos*-kinship world of status relations to the *polis* world of transactions consummated under the rule of law," a moment when earlier Indo-European variety in marriage relations was reduced in Athens to a single form of marriage.[5] The legal transformation was accompanied by a change in the gifts conveyed: Homeric *hedna* was effaced by dowry, to which Homeric Greek had earlier affixed no standard name, but which was now called sometimes *proix,* more frequently *pherne.*[6] Many scholars would similarly deny that Roman *coemptio* ever resembled marriage by purchase in which bridewealth was conveyed and, in spite of the silence of the XII Tables, would argue that Roman marriage was always dotal.[7] If not a legal requirement for the match, as it became in Greece, the Roman dowry nevertheless seems early on to have rendered the marriage respectable: the Plautine figure Trinummus worried "lest the word would be passed round that I gave you my sister for a concubine if I give her without dowry."[8]

Whether it gradually disappeared or had never existed, the historical absence of brideprice in Greece and Rome demarcated Greco-Roman society not only from contemporary Indo-European peoples such as the Celts and Germans but also from most of the ancient and historic peoples of the Mediterranean, whose legal and religious literature, from the Code of Hammurabi to the Bible, records their practice of brideprice.[9] Yet there are signs that brideprice almost inevitably began to wane as those ancient Mediterranean civilizations grew and flourished, and perhaps Greco-Roman practice merely enshrined a pattern that was becoming established in the Mediterranean. Although Old Babylonian myths concentrate on the gifts borne by a bridegroom to the house of his bride, for example, some gift lists suggest a more varied and balanced exchange. Furthermore, the Code of Hammurabi (art. 164) already envisioned a dowry [*seriktu*] whose worth would generally exceed the brideprice [*tirhatu*], which later law and contracts suggest may have fallen out of use.[10] So, too, in ancient Egypt brideprice seems first to have been displaced by a husband's gift to the bride and then, in the sixth century when a new type of marriage arose, by a gift conveyed by the bride herself.[16,11]

It is a distinction that still sets the Mediterranean apart. Practised by only four percent of the cultures analyzed in Murdoch's *World Ethnographic Atlas,* dotal marriage is limited geographically to eastern Eurasia and to the Mediterranean, upon whose shores its hold is most secure.[12] Thus dotal marriage may be both a synchronic and diachronic sign of the much-heralded unity and distinctiveness of Mediterranean culture. But like the related if more notorious complex of honor and shame, anthropological study of its synchrony has not been matched by adequate historical inquiry into its past. Hence, apart from the belief, which is at least as old as Aristotle, that dotal marriage is the product of a beneficial evolution toward higher civilization, the reasons for its adoption within the Mediterranean remain essentially mysterious and the process of change from brideprice to dowry is virtually unknown.

The question is complex. Brideprice and dowry are not, as Goody has repeatedly stressed, opposite or opposed gifts; they can and frequently do coexist. The Babylonian case is a clear example of this, but so, too, is that of the Hebrews, who seem—like almost all of the Semitic and Indo-European races—to have awarded their daughters a gift to take into marriage even though the central and legally required settlement long remained the brideprice [*môhar*][13] Nor are brideprice and dowry the only awards conveyed at marriage. Goody has drawn attention to a third category of gift, which he terms indirect dowry and which passes from the bridegroom to the bride.[14] Strabo speaks of the Cantabrians whose husbands gave dowries [*proixa*] to their brides, who would bequeath them to their daughters, an apposite institution, he felt, in a society dominated by its women. But the Babylonians knew *nudunnu* (Code of Hammurabi, arts. 171-2), and a similar award may be found in Ptolemaic Egypt.[15] And there are other awards as well: gifts, apart from the brideprice, taken by the groom into the house of the bride—the *biblu* of the Babylonians, the *mathon* of the Hebrews, perhaps the *hedna* of the Homeric Greeks—or gifts given to the bride herself, such as the offering made after the consummation of the marriage in recognition of her virginity, an award that has often escaped historical notice because it usually had no legal status. We would not know of its presence in dotal Rome if Juvenal, in his biting satire on marital chastity, had not wondered, "Why lose a salver of newly-minted gold pieces—victory issues, at that—on the first-night bridal offering?" (VI:203-4).

It is often difficult, both historically and ethnologically, to single out the central or binding gifts to construct a series of "systems" or patterns of change. But it seems important to notice that within many of the civilizations that have imprinted their customs on the lands of the Mediterranean gifts awarded by bridegrooms to wives or their kinsmen tended to become overshadowed by the settlement from her own family that the bride carried to her husband's home. This settlement, or dowry, universal though its presence was, showed important qualitative and quantitative variations. Among the Hebrews, for example, it remained the woman's property; among the Greeks, her husband managed it during the marriage; at Rome, in a marriage with *manus,* it originally fell totally into the husband's control. So, too, in some places it might consist of a small trousseau, in others a considerable settlement by a woman's family that represented her effective share of the patrimony. Both its quality and its value will, of course, tend to shape any system of which dowry forms a part. It seems clear, however, that Greco-Roman society knew dotal marriage, both in the sense that gifts from the groom were minimal or trivial and in the sense that the dowry tended to be a weighty and substantial settlement on which prospective bridegrooms might cast greedy eyes.[16] It is hard to know whether the Greeks and Romans were the first to arrive at this full dotal state, but they have left the fullest account of how that system worked. Unfortunately Greco-Roman sources do not take us far toward understanding why they came to adopt and develop this form of marriage.

Perhaps the ancient world will never give up those secrets, but it is possible to study the Mediterranean predilection for dowry from the vantage point of a later, better-documented period—that of the early Middle Ages, from the time of the Germanic invasions of the fifth century, which shattered this uniquely dotal world that the Greeks and Romans had created.[17] The weight of Germanic settlement in this period imposed on large areas of the western Mediterranean a system of marital pretestations, the chief of which was not a dowry bestowed by father on daughter but the husband's donation that Tacitus described. Although, as we shall see, the custom of granting dowry to daughters may have been retained by some of the

Roman population while an analogous gift gained ground even within German communities, the important and binding marriage settlement came almost everywhere to be the husband's gift. A Constitution of 458 of the emperor Majoran had briefly made dowry necessary for legal marriage within the crumbling Empire, news of which a letter of Pope Leo carried so effectively throughout the West that the phrase "Nullum sine dote fiat conjugium" (Let there be no marriage without dowry) became a commonplace in early medieval laws and charters. In them, however, it referred not to Roman dowry but to the husband's gift. It was this gift alone that Pope Nicholas I mentioned in his letter of 866 in which he outlined to the Bulgarians the form of marriage current among Latin Christians in the West.[18]

Yet within five centuries of is demise, the dowry had begun to re-emerge; and the hiatus produced by the invasions was forgotten.[19] The cities that grew and prospered on the northern shore of the Mediterranean in the High Middle Ages, like those of the classical world, were dotal cities. Indeed when Renaissance Italian cities began to feel the pinch of dowries, they looked to the classical world as the source of both the problem and its remedy: Memmo called for their abolition in Venice, where, according to a law of 1537, youth "no longer do business in the city or go to sea. . .placing all hope in extravagant dowry;"[20] and he cited as his authority Lycurgus, who had supposedly solved ancient Sparta's problems by banning dowries there.[21]

Fortunately this millennium of change can be studied in some detail through two kinds of fairly full and abundant documentation: laws and charters. Into the first category fall both the superb legal codes and collections of late imperial Rome and the more difficult and incomplete compilations of law and custom issued by Germanic rulers, ecclesiastical and feudal law, customary law, and urban statutes. In the second category we can place all documents of practice, from the single, often cryptic charters of the early Middle Ages to the rich notarial chartularies of the medieval and Renaissance city. Such documentation is, of course, not evenly distributed. Legal evidence must dominate the earliest period, up until about the eighth century, when it begins to be complemented by charters; but it is only from about the twelfth century that the richness of documents of practice lets us compare statutory norms and social behavior.[22] Used with care, however, these sources let us come to a reasonably full understanding of the changes in the system of marital assigns that occurred in the western Mediterranean during the Middle Ages. Perhaps they can also contribute to the current search for both a general theory of marital assigns and a more refined knowledge of the history of the cultural institutions of the Mediterranean.

II

Germanic marriage, like marriage almost everywhere, wove a web of gifts and settlements of which we can still observe only the most substantial and enduring strands. Giftgiving, as Mauss has shown, is a way of exerting power, which the Germanic recipient had traditionally both to acknowledge and to counteract by awarding a formal and obligatory countergift.[23] Even the marital arrangements that Tacitus briefly described had about them this flavor of guarded exchange; for after the groom gave his bride those gifts so clearly designed for her kinsmen's eyes, she bestowed on him a small countergift, "some present of arms."[24] Here, however, I shall concern myself with only the three major Germanic assigns: brideprice, a payment made by a groom to his wife's kinsmen in return for their relinquishing control of her *mundium,* a legal guardianship or protection exercised in Germanic society over women and other incompetents before the law; morning gift [*morgengabe*], a groom's payment to his bride the morning after the consummation of their marriage as the price of, or reward for, her virginity; and, finally, the father's gift that daughters might receive when they left their natal home to marry.

Tacitus' failure to mention brideprice[25] may indicate that even by the end of the first century it had fallen from prominence among those tribes that lived on the fringes of the Empire. Certainly by the time these West German tribes issued their law codes, brideprice had generally disappeared. Thus the Alamannic, Thuringian, and Frankish codes legislate concerning a husband's gift to the bride but are silent about brideprice paid to her kinsmen. But Frankish literary and formulary evidence indicates that in the traditional one solidus and one denarius paid by Frankish grooms to the fathers of their brides, we should see the vestigial remains of a brideprice that had probably once been paid by all West Germans. This assumption is strengthened by the example of the Saxons, a West German people who were exceptional in the length of their migrations and whose law code, redacted as late as the ninth century, records a brideprice fixed as equal to the legal worth of the bride, to her *wergeld.*[26]

The tribes that invaded, settled, and transformed the northern shore of the Mediterranean, however, were not descendants of those whose customs Tacitus purported to record. They were almost wholly Scandinavian or East German tribes, whose migrations tended to be late and long. All of their legal codes mention brideprice; and they show its tendency to change from a payment made to kinsmen of the bride to a donation made to the bride herself. The Burgundians, who after a long migration from Scandinavia to the Vistula and west into the Empire settled finally in southeastern Gaul in the fifth century, seem to have awarded one-third of their brideprice [*wittimon*] to their wives, two-thirds to their wives' kinsmen. Among the Visigoths, who made themselves masters of southwestern France and the Iberian peninsula after a similar migration, an ancient brideprice seems to have been totally incorporated in the award that grooms made to their brides by the time the law codes were issued.[27] The Lombards, a people whose origins, though perhaps Scandinavian, still remain obscure,[28] may still have awarded brideprice [*meta*] to their wives' kinsmen in the seventh century when Rothair issued his Edict; but half a century later, under King Liutprand, the wives themselves regularly received it.[29] Perhaps even in Rothair's day it was customary for the woman's parents to bestow the *meta* upon their daughters, much as Penelope's may have done: a twelfth-century marriage charter from southern Italy in which a groom promised a certain sum as "meffio" to his father-in-law, who then turned it over to the daughter-bride, seems to capture in petrified form a transmutation of *meta* which occurred after the Lombards had settled on the Italian peninsula but which their laws do not fully record.[30]

Change in direction of brideprice signals a change in its character. In both Saxon and Lombard evidence, brideprice was a compensation paid to a woman's kinsmen in exchange for control of the woman herself or of her *mundium.* The redirection of brideprice toward the woman and away from her kin is undoubtedly a sign that any real sense of exchange had begun to fade. Among the Visigoths, for example, the law allowed women remarkable freedom in selecting a husband.[31] And even where kinsmen continued to convey her *mundium* to her husband, this conveyance was no longer what gave marriage legitimacy among the Germans. Rothair's Edict already recognized the case of marriage in which the husband "neglected to acquire [his wife's] *mundium*" (188), and popular Germanic custom seems eventually to have allowed as perfectly legal, if perhaps somewhat unusual, marriages in which the husband never secured control of the *mundium* of his wife.[32]

What came to replace the transfer of *mundium* as the mark of a legal marriage was the formal act of consummation, recognized by the gift that would dominate Germanic prestations in the historic age, the morning gift. Unlike brideprice, which almost everywhere had shrunk to a modest or symbolic gift, *morgengabe* remained a substantial and meaningful assign, like the five cities that Gregory of Tours tells us the Merovingian king Chilperic awarded his bride Galsuntha, sister of the fierce Brunhilda, "tam in dote quam in morganegyba hoc est matutinale donum." Even outside court circles the assign was important among West Germans. The Ripuarian Code informs us, for example, that among these Franks a traditional, customary morning gift was 50 solidi. This represented a quarter of the *wergeld* of a freeman or the price of 25 oxen.[33]

But it is the tribes that imprinted their customs on the Mediterranean that have left the fullest and most revealing records of *morgengabe.* Its clearest description is contained in the law codes and formulas of the Visigoths and Lombards. The Burgundian Code is less explicit, regulating only the wife's usufruct rights in her morning gift [*donatio nuptialis*],[34] whose importance the literary imagination preserved, however, in countless stories of the awful treasure of the Nibelungs:

> Kriemhild sent 800 men to fetch it from where it lay hidden and where Alberic with his nearest kinsmen guarded it. When they saw the men of the Rhine come for the treasure, bold Alberic spoke to his friends, "We dare not refuse her the treasure, for it is the noble queen's morning gift". . . . Now hear the marvels of this treasure. Twelve wagons could scarcely carry it there in four days and four nights although each of them made the journey three times. It was all precious stones and gold, and had the whole of the world been bought with it, it would not have been in the least diminished. . . [35]

Both Lombard and Visigothic *morgengabe* seem also to have been initially conveyed in moveable wealth. The Visigothic king Chindasvind, for example, in legislation designed to limit the morning gift among his people, allowed to nobles [*primates palatii*], in addition to a substantial money grant, ten slave boys, ten slave girls, and twenty horses; and a verse formula from the reign of his predecessor suggests that these were the goods in which the traditional Visigothic *morgengabe* was conveyed:

> Lo we give you first ten boys and an equal number of girls, ten horses and an equal number of mules; and further we grant arms, for such is the ancient morgingeba of the Goths.[36]

In both the Visigothic and Lombard kingdoms, moreover, the morning gift increased in value as its nature began also to change. The donation of landed wealth along with the traditional *morgengabe* appears in the earliest Visigothic formulas; and an enumeration in 739 of the *morgengabe* of a dead woman from Lucca includes not only slaves, furniture, and clothes, but also houses.[37] The proportion of property conveyed seems to have grown until men at marriage awarded their wives substantial parts of their real property. King Chindasvind's legislation fixed a ceiling of one-tenth of a man's estate on marriage grants to wives, which had earlier risen to include as much as one-half of the husband's worth.[38] King Reccesvind extended the limit in 681 by allowing, in addition to the ancient morgengabe and Chindasvind's tenth, a grant of 1000 solidi, a sum which Chindasvind's legislation had earlier equated with the tenth of the richest Visigoths.[39] Later charters from the Iberian peninsula show that this combination became traditional. In one from 887, for instance, a certain Sisnandus declared:

> I give and concede to you my dear spouse as your dower [in titulum dotis] 10 boys: these are Fromarigius, Petrus, Betotus, Recaredus, Malulus, Feles, Marcitus, Egela, Severinus, Lopellus; so too 10 girls: these are Teodosinda, Maluca, Egilo, Gonza, Rosalia, Domnina, Guncina, Oihenia, Ansoi, Piniola; 20 horses, and a mule with saddle and ornamented bridle, 50 [more] horses . . ., 100 cows, 20 yoke of oxen, 500 mixed animals, 400 solidi in ornaments and clothes, 30 villas . . . and, over and above that, one-tenth of all my goods.[40]

In Italy, King Liutprand was trying to establish its limits in 717 when he legislated that *morgengabe* could not exceed one-quarter of a man's worth;[41] and, as among the Visigoths, the ceiling quickly became a tradition, making *quarta* the customary Lombard wedding gift.

Both Visigothic *decima* and Lombard *quarta* resembled a contemporary Frankish and Burgundian institution, the dower which awarded widows usufruct rights in a portion of their husbands' estates. Among the Burgundians, for example, in addition to her "morgenegiva," a childless widow received one-third of her husband's property.[42] Similarly, and perhaps through Burgundian influence, the Ripuarian Law allowed to widows who had not received a written dower from their husbands 50 solidi in cash and one-third of all increase in the estate from the time of the marriage, a right to a portion of the acquisitions that came to be extended to all widows.[43] A Capitulary of 821, for example, gave all Frankish widows a claim to one-third of the benefices that their husbands had acquired in the course of the marriage.[44] And by the ninth century, this third had come to pertain to the whole of the Frankish husband's estate.[45] A marriage formula from Lombard Italy, which had absorbed large numbers of Franks in the Carolingian period, stipulated that a man living under Salic, that is Frankish, law was to dower his wife with one-third [*tercia*] of all his present goods and future acquisitions. Another supplied a standard form with two simple substitutions to cover the award of the husband's gift throughout the peninsula: the Roman or Salic husband had only to replace the Lombard "morgincap" with "carta dotis" and, "de quarta portione" of the Lombards with "de tercia portione" of the Franks.[46]

Throughout most Christian communities of the western Mediterranean, then, *morgengabe* with its associated portion had come to assure brides—both Roman and Germanic—of substantial rights in the patrimonies of their husbands: over one-tenth in Spain and western France, one-quarter in the Lombard areas of Italy, and one-third wherever Frankish and Burgundian custom held sway. Women's control of their portion varied—certainly from one area to another, probably too among social groups (although charters, which overwhelmingly record aristocratic practice, are less help here). As childless widows their immediate claim to morning gift is everywhere unmistakable. The Alamannic widow could say,

> "My husband gave me the morginaghapha." She should compute what it was in silver, gold or in slaves or in horses. . . . Then she can swear on her breast and say, "That my husband gave me to control, and I should have it."[47]

Among the Alamanni, *morgengabe,* like the alternative *dotis legitima,* may have fallen quite fully into her control.[48] Most German brides, however, seem to have had legally and in the presence of children only rights of usufruct over the grant. The Burgundian widow who remarried might have her *morgengabe* only in usufruct. She could not "give, sell, or transfer what she received in this gift [*donatio*]," and after her death her sons received it all. Only Visigothic law was more generous; in addition to the usufruct in a share of the estate equal to that of each of her children, a widow was allowed to dispose freely of one-quarter of her husband's gift [*dos*] and one-fifth of any "extradotal" gift he might have awarded her (IV:5.2; V:2.4).[49]

There are many indications, however, that by the ninth and tenth centuries a wife's claim on her marriage portion had grown stronger throughout the western Mediterranean. Perhaps she might not be generally so free with it as Kriemhild, who, when she

> got it into her keeping . . . gave more freely than ever had been seen. To poor and rich did she begin to give, til Hagen said that if she lived but a while longer, she would win so many knights to her service that it must go hard with the others. King Gunther said, "It is her own. How she uses it does not concern me. . ." But Hagen said to the king, "A wise man would leave such treasure to no woman"[50]

But many men ignored such counsel; and a widow's right to alienate at least part of her morning gift gained currency and took customary form in large areas of southern Europe. In Burgundy, for example, some husbands exploited the composite nature of the husband's gift to award specific rights of full ownership to their wives. In widowhood these women exercised proprietorship over a particular assigned gift, which may have been related to the ancient donation of *morgengabe* in moveable goods, but enjoyed only rights of usufruct over their portion.[51] This is the clear implication of the two gifts that the Burgundian Ermengerius made in 912 to his bride Dotana. By one charter he awarded her "in *mergingiva* according to my law of Gundobad" specific property in several locations to do with as she chose; by a second, he conferred on her as "dotalicium" usufruct of the traditional Burgundian third of his estate.[52]

Almost everywhere, even in the absence of such refinements, the claim of widows to ownership of their *morgengabe* had begun to edge out the traditional inheritance rights of their husbands' kinsmen. The Visigothic law was exceptional in allowing childless widows free disposition of their husbands' gifts. Other codes were more severe: among the Burgundians all of the portion and half of the *morgengabe* returned to her husband's heirs; among the Lombards they received it all. His kinsmen's hostility to the reduction of their rights may be why in Burgundy in 909 a certain Fulcherius promised his wife, before an assembly of her kinsmen, that his relatives could not cancel her ownership of the 100 estates and 50 serfs that he had just awarded her "in sponsalitium." Even in Lombard Italy, where hostility to women's property rights was particularly strong, widows—like Atta who in 927 sold goods that she had received through charters of "donatio" and "morgincap" from her late husband—more than occasionally managed to alienate their morning gifts.[53]

A woman's rights as the wife of a living husband are harder to assess. In Spain, where marriage charters frequently granted wives full freedom over their morning gift from the moment of its donation, women seem in practice to have exercised considerable control over property; and although a causal connection has by no means been established, some evidence suggests that both there and elsewhere in southern Europe married women frequently managed their marital assigns.[54] Many Burgundian charters state unequivocally that the wife can treat her marriage gift as she chooses. Even a particularly flowery one composed for a certain Eldebertus when he decided in 833 to obey the will of God, who "to produce a multitude of children, ordained the union [*copulationem*] of men and women, saying 'Increase and multiply and fill the land,' " is down to earth concerning the right of his new bride to "sell, donate, or commute" the property he conferred upon her. It may be the full identification of Burgundian women with the property they received as morning gifts that forced one husband to acknowledge a flaw in the gift: one of the serfs he awarded his wife was a rascal [*cattivo*]—but, he hastened to add, sound in mind and body.[55] And even in Italy restrictions imposed by Lombard legal incapacity apparently did not prevent some wives from exercising control over their marriage gifts.[56]

Perhaps more commonly the Germanic morning gift, as it developed in the ninth and tenth centuries on the northern shore of the Mediterranean, encouraged association between husbands and the wives to whom they had granted a portion of their landed wealth. Burgues has seen tendencies in this direction in Languedoc where it began to lead to an effective association of conjugal goods. And the regularity, both in Burgundy and in Lombard Italy, with which wives were called to consent to their husbands' sales and alienations suggests that *tercia* and *quarta* gave them a considerable role in the management of the conjugal estate.[57]

At the same time, the woman's contribution may have grown more extensive. Germanic fathers did often award their daughters a gift when they left home to marry, the so-called *faderfio.* This was the splendid gift that King Chilperic's daughter carried with her into Spain for her marriage. Her father, staggered by its size, feared that it had emptied the royal treasury. Although the queen had, by her own admission, contributed considerable of her personal wealth to the girl, it seems clear that the largest part of the "gold and silver and other ornaments" that filled 50 wagons came from her *faderfio.*[58]

In both Visigothic Spain and Lombard Italy, the father's gift, perhaps initially no more than a modest trousseau, grew in prominence and in substance during the seventh and eighth centuries. The provision in Spain that the maximum *morgengabe* of one-tenth might be exceeded if the surplus was matched by an equivalent gift from the wife may have encouraged its expansion. King Rothair recognized it already in the eighth century as a serious gift which Lombard husbands had come to anticipate. In King Liutprand's day, some Lombard daughters might receive as *faderfio* as much as one-quarter of the paternal estate.[59] Although in both Spain and Italy, a daughter's claim at marriage to a share of her paternal inheritance may have been strengthened through analogy with dowries given within the Roman population, the *faderfio* differed from Roman dowry in at least one important way; it was not legally required for a marriage, and it never formed part of the marriage charter.[60]

Among the Roman population of the South, dowry probably never disappeared. Benedict of Soratte recalls in his tenth-century chronicle that

> [the eighth-century Lombard king] Ratchis took a wife called Tassia, a woman from the city of Rome, and broke his native Lombard law by not giving the morgyncaph and methio that it required. Instead he made donations by Roman charter as the

> Romans asked. For this the Lombards were enraged and, treating with Aistulf about his kingdom, drove out King Ratchis . . .[61]

Throughout Italy dowry remained the prevalent marriage settlement in many Byzantine areas, and scholars have found hints of continued dotal presence elsewhere on the peninsula.[62] But even in Italy no known marriage settlement actually mentions the Roman dowry. For Romans as well as Germans, marriage seems to have come to revolve around the husband's gift. According to a Carolingian formula for the donation of morning gift in Lombard Italy *(above p. 22),* men who lived by Roman law awarded their wives the Frankish *tercia;* and contemporary charters show that this was a common practice within some parts of Italy. At Pavia in 921, for instance, a husband living by Roman law promised to secure his wife rights to one-third of his estate. But some Roman wives received the Lombard *quarta,* in which they may have recognized a resemblance to the claim of one-quarter of a husband's estate that Justinian had allowed poor widows.[63]

More generally they may have seen in the Roman counterdower an institution with similarities to the Germanic husband's gift. This originally small countergift to the dowry, which some would see as a survival of ancient Roman bridewealth, had so increased in value by the third century that its worth sometimes exceeded the dowry.[64] It was this abuse that the emperor Majoran tried to correct by equalizing dowry and countergift. In so doing, he attacked the cupidity of Roman brides and their families, who, by extracting extravagant counterdowers from their grooms, were devouring their substance, forcing marriages to be delayed, and thus lowering the birthrate. Some women apparently paid their dowries from the counterdower and thus effectively contributed nothing to the match.[65] It may have been such fraudulent practices that prompted Majoran to proclaim "Nullum sine dote fiat conjugium," the sentiment that gained such undeserved currency in the medieval West. The rise in the value of the Roman counterdower (called the *donatio propter nuptias* after the time of Justinian, who finally established its equivalence with the dowry) and its at least occasional conversion from a credit to a real grant suggest that on the eve of the Germanic invasions, even in the heart of the Empire, husbands had begun to pay.

In general, then, the population of the western Mediterranean in the early Middle Ages, no matter what its ethnic origin, had adopted a system of marital assigns whose chief award was neither the dowry of the ancient world nor the brideprice of the ancient Germans but a grant that had grown out of *morgengabe,* originally awarded to the wife as the price of her virginity. That formal recognition of a wife's virginity retained extraordinary force and resonance within aristocratic society in the early Middle Ages, as the chronical by Hincmar of Reims relating the endless marital struggle between Lothair II of Lotharingia and his wife Teutberga shows. Teutberga, the daughter of Boso of Burgundy, married Lothair in 857. Her misfortune was twofold: she did not bear a child, and she could not replace in her husband's affections his former concubine Waldrada, whom he shortly decided he would like to marry. As grounds for divorce, Lothair charged Teutberga with incestuous sodomy with her brother, who, he claimed had made her pregnant before their marriage—although this had gone undetected at the time because the queen had aborted the fetus. Teutberga wholeheartedly denied this, of course; but what may have thwarted Lothair's ambitions—at least temporarily—was a public admission he had made of Teutberga's virginity through his grant of *morgengabe.*[66] Certainly a few years later Pope Nicholas was to argue against him that he would not allow a marriage to be dissolved if, after consummating the match and paying the husband's gift, the husband discovered that his wife had not been a virgin. Nicholas would go further to forbid almost any grounds for divorce, but it may have been the claims and counterclaims concerning Lothair's nuptual gifts that sparked Hincmar's interest in the case; for he was drawn to the support of *morgengabe* as the test of a valid marriage.[67]

In Visigothic Spain marriage charters continued to specify into the tenth and eleventh centuries that husbands conferred their marriage gift "in acknowledgement of virginity." In Lombard Tuscany Algozo di Bonizone might set out in a charter in November 1029 the contents of the "moriincap" he would award his future bride Julla: one quarter of all his estates in the countryside around Arezzo, including castles and churches, serfs and slaves, animals and arms "according to our law of the Lombards." But he was required formally to confirm the gift before their relatives on the day after the marriage when the union had been consummated (quando te mihi a coinio copulavero). Even in Byzantine Venice, which continued its dotal course almost uninterrupted, the traditional counterassign to dowry was not the *donatio propter nuptias* of Justinian's Code but a

"Monday gift" [*donum dei lunae*] offered the day after the wedding (and so-named because of the Venetian practice of celebrating marriage on Sunday), which seems to have retained its characteristic association with the price of virginity.[68]

Customary *morgengabe* made room for exceptions: widows seem generally to have received it, for example.[69] Rather than calling it a *pretium virginitatis,* it is perhaps better to see it as a man's formal claim to sexual rights over his wife—no longer purchased from her kin, but gained from the woman herself. Both the economic and legal qualities of *morgengabe* stressed relations between the marital couple at the expense of the kinsmen whose authority brideprice had recognized. Rape or abduction had been regularized among the Germans by a payment of brideprice or a multiple of it to the woman's kin;[70] but as brideprice everywhere lost its value and significance, that compensation tended to disappear. It was now not her kin but the woman herself to whom payment was directed. Thus in the early Middle Ages rape could be turned into marriage by the payment of *morgengabe.*[71] The morning gift can, finally, stand as a symbol of a new, medieval view of marriage. Marriage was based neither on the consent of the parties, as it had been in Rome, nor on the conveyal of rights through purchase, as it had been earlier among the Germans. Instead attention focused on the sexual act. Recognition of a real relationship in blood established by sexual intercourse underlay the Church's early extension of the incest prohibition to include those with whom an individual—or his kin or affines—had ever had carnal relations.[72] And while it is certainly true that the husband's gift, as it evolved through the centuries in the West, was often awarded before the marriage was consummated, the validity of the gift could be called into question if such consummation did not follow: the Customs of Tortosa denied a husband's gift to wives whose husbands had died before they had consummated the marriage.[73] In the early Middle Ages formal consummation made a marriage, and *morgengabe* was its sign.

III

By the thirteenth century the world had changed. There came before the court of the archbishop in Pisa on 7 July 1230 the case between Bonfiliolus and Benvenuta, who refused to live with him as his wife because, she claimed, at the time of their engagement he already had a wife called Ugolina. Bonfiliolus retorted that he had never taken Ugolina as his wife. But, fearing death at the hands of her kinsmen, he had given her a ring. Moreover, he showed the court Benvenuta's dotal charter as proof that *she* was his wife. Force in the one case, the presence of dowry in the other, led the court to declare valid his marriage with Benvenuta—a Roman world of dowry and consent.[74]

Dowry began to re-emerge in Italy, southern France, and Catalonia in about the eleventh century in the wake of peace, economic and demographic growth, and the establishment of public authority; and within two centuries it had successfully reestablished itself as the chief marital assign of the Mediterranean littoral.[75] Its rise coincided everywhere with the decline of the customary morning gift, whose nature became strictly usufructual and whose value was ultimately pegged to the dowry. In the countryside around Mâcon, in Burgundy, in and around Marseille, in Provence, and in the city of Montpellier, in Languedoc, grants of specific property ceased to form part of the morning gift, which became in the eleventh and twelfth centuries only a guarantee to the widow of usufruct rights in a portion of her husband's estate.[76] In Catalonia and in Italy, where the process of change is clearly documented, restrictions on the morning gift represent attempts to preserve the integrity of an estate by keeping control over strategic property out of the hands of wives and widows. In Barcelona, for instance, marriage charters of the twelfth century had begun to stipulate that in the event of the husband's death his kinsmen could purchase for a specified sum property that had been granted as "sponsalitium." Thus Mir de Mollet arranged in 1170 that if his wife Guilerma should outlive him, his relatives might repurchase the fief he had granted as her marriage gift for 800 morabiti of gold; and the 1193 marriage charter of Berenguer set a repurchase price of 300 morabiti on the *sponsalitium* he gave his wife Arsenda.[77]

In Italy attempts to exclude strategic property from grants of *quarta* and *tercia* seem to have encouraged an early abolition of the donation itself. A priest making donation of all his goods in the territory of Milan in 1090 stipulated that in future no woman might have the Lombard *quarta* of his fortress (*castrum*); less than a century later in Vercelli a husband living by Frankish law had, perhaps under parental force, denied his wife *tercia* in churches and fortresses, a restriction he eventually revoked in 1171. In 1187 in the territory of Piedmont a certain Alaisius made a convenant with his wife Talia that should he die without heirs she would take no *quarta* from his goods. Throughout Lombardy *quarta* was seen as a threat to feudal order and property control. The Milanese customal of 1216, recording a practice that may have been a century old, states that "A woman should only have *quarta* from private property, and not from rented or feudal lands", while expressing in general its "abhorrence of *quarta.*"[78] Yet it seems that Lombard cities were reluctant to extend their prohibition to abolition. Bergamo and Brescia, for example, also forbade *quarta* in feudal lands, but let the donation remain.[79] The earliest complete abolition of the Germanic portion came not in its Lombard heartland but in Liguria, where by a consular decree issued in Genoa in 1143, customary *tercia* was forbidden in the future and, except for widows who were already in possession, present grants were annulled.[80] The dismay of the city's women—captured in the illustration that adorns Genoa's contemporary annals of two of their number, hands upraised in protest or despair[81]—had no practical effects. The series of notarial chartularies that begins slightly more than a decade after the decree contains only one mention of *tercia;* and this undoubtedly refers to a widow who was already in possession before 1143.[82] One Italian city after another followed Genoa's lead until, by the middle of the thirteenth century, in no major commune in northern Italy could women expect to receive the Germanic portion.[83]

After 1143 Genoese women were allowed only a smaller counterdower, their so-called *antefactum* (or *donatio propter nuptias*), which was itself reduced from the dotal equality recommended by Justinian to a value not in excess of half the dowry, or 100 Genoese pounds, whichever was smaller. Other cities placed similar limitations on this assign. Generally set as one-half or one-quarter of the woman's dowry, it was everywhere only a credit that she could claim as a widow. In many cities, wives could claim the *donatio* only under special conditions: if the marriage had produced no sons, for example, or if the husband had made special provisions in his will.[84]

Other Mediterranean cities, in a less formal way, followed the Italian example of abolishing the Germanic marriage portion and allowing only a modest counterdower. At Toulouse, for example, the portion had disappeared by the fourteenth century, when the city's brides received from their husbands only a "don de noces," a credit that was commonly worth one-half or one-third of their dowry. So too, a *sponsalitium* that had represented usufruct of one-half of the husband's estate in twelfth-century Montpellier was replaced in the following century by a dotal augment [*augmentum dotis*] that seldom attained even half the worth of the woman's dowry; and by the end of the fourteenth century, the augment had been reduced to a traditional gift of predictably small size, tied neither to the worth of the dowry nor to that of the husband's estate.[85]

Although scattered references show that the traditional Visigothic tenth was still alive in Catalonia in the thirteenth century, in Barcelona[86] it was superseded by the *sponsalitium,* an assign of settled and substantial value. The *sponsalitium,* which may have descended from the part of the *morgengabe* that had consisted of specific goods, was generally composed of assigned lands or other real estate, like the house and vineyard outside the city's walls that Marti Petit awarded his spouse in 1116. But it could also be awarded in cash, as was the *sponsalitium* of 400 gold mancusi that Eg received from her husband Bernard Udalard in 1100.[87] Sometimes the wife exercised only rights of usufruct over her *sponsalitium,* which after her death descended to her children or, in their absence, to her husband's heirs. But frequently she was awarded rights of ownership over one-half (or more) of the grant. Thus Raimon Gombaldi gave to his wife Stephania in 1209 full ownership of 700 solidi from her 1200 solidi *sponsalitium.*[88] By the end of the thirteenth century, however, the *sponsalitium* had disappeared. In its place the wives of Barcelona began to receive a dotal augment, the *escreix.* The Custom of Tortosa prescribed an *escreix* of one-half the value of the dowry contributed by the wife, and such an arrangement may have been traditional throughout Catalonia. It was certainly customary in Barcelona until at least the end of the fourteenth century.[89] Although a wife was occasionally given ownership rights in part of her *escreix,* its more usual form was a grant in usufruct that returned at her death to their children or to her husband's heirs.[90] The *escreix,* then, like the augment in Montpellier or the *antefactum* in Genoa, was a grant clearly inferior to the Germanic portion or its close descendants. Still, the Catalonian counterdower seemed extravagant to some husbands: when in 1299 a certain Suavis married in Barcelona and gave as her dowry the entirety of her maternal inheritance bolstered by an additional cash grant of 260 solidi, her husband balked at an *escreix* of even half the cash, giving instead a meager amount of 80 solidi.[91] But, then, although a citizen of Barcelona, he had come from Italy—where men paid even less dear.

Throughout the world of the western Mediterranean, women

were coming to depend far less on the generosity of their husbands than on that of their own kin, whose award of a dowry became a prerequisite of marriage, the burdens of which it was held to sustain. Dowry has been called premortem inheritance, in which a daughter's share of her father's estate is served up early, when she needs it to enter and establish a new home, rather than at the time of her father's death.[92] Both the governments and jurists of the medieval Mediterranean stressed the close relation between dowry and female inheritance rights, even though such a stand was, in a sense, contrary to the tenets of Roman law, whose adoption throughout southern Europe had undoubtedly encouraged the spread of dotal practice.[93] In communal Italy the view of dowry as a substitute for a daughter's normal claim on her father's estate is at least as old as the Pisan *constitutum usus,* redacted between 1140 and 1144, which denied to dowered daughters further rights in their paternal inheritance, a principle that became enshrined in the statutes of a sufficient number of communes to become a general rule in northern Italy.[94] The exclusion may have found its source in a statement by the Lombard king Rothair that a bridegroom must be content with the portion of her father's or mother's estate brought by his bride at the time of their marriage. This was a position that had been annulled by Liutprand's decree that married and unmarried daughters were to inherit equally;[95] but the provision of Rothair's Edict may well have continued to have practical force in Lombard Italy. Yet it cannot be attributed solely to Lombard attitudes, for it caught on almost everywhere. In Provence, where in the eleventh and early twelfth centuries daughters seem often to have shared the same familial rights as sons, almost exactly contemporary statutes began to exclude dowered daughters. At Arles a statute of about 1150 denied to "daughters dowered by their fathers or their mothers" any further claim on their paternal or maternal estate, a proscription transferred four years later into the charter that Avignon received from its bishop; and by the thirteenth century the exclusion had swept through the rest of southern France.[96] In Catalonia the association of dowry with female inheritance rights can be traced as far back as a document of 988 in which a certain Oddo awarded dowry [*exovar*] to his daughter "as the inheritance you should inherit from me."[97] Principles of Visigothic and Roman law may have served in Catalonia, even more than in Provence, to encourage equality among children; but wills show that by the end of the twelfth century a dowry was beginning to be seen as a daughter's final claim on the estate. Guillermo Pere de Sarriá provided in his will of 1148, for example, that if his son Berengerius married off his two sisters honorably, he might receive the legacies that Guillermo provided for their dowries.[98] In Catalonia a woman's dowry came, at least by the fourteenth century, to be the *only* portion of the paternal estate to which she had legitimate claim.[99]

The extent of the exclusion was not everywhere the same. Although dowered daughters were always excluded from intestate succession in the presence of sons of the deceased, their rights with respect to brothers were less certain: in Provence the daughters' claims were recognized as superior, but in neighboring Liguria uncles preceded them.[100] In Genoa numerous fathers did, in the absence of sons or grandsons, exclude brothers in their wills to secure the estate for their married daughters; but this was an essentially popular practice that did not begin to make headway among the city's patriciate until late in the fourteenth century.[101] In many places, furthermore, dotal exclusion had an unmistakable flavor of masculine privilege; for it excluded dowered women not only from the estate of the person who had dowered them but also from the more extensive family estate. The precise ingredients of such exclusion varied, perhaps in accordance with the needs of familial organization. In the cities of Provence, for example, dowered daughters were excluded rigorously from the narrow conjugal group: they could not inherit from their fathers, mothers, sisters, or brothers. But they were not kept from the succession of grandparents or more distant collaterals.[102] In Genoa, as perhaps in Forcalquier, lineage took precedence over household to narrow the group from whose succession dowered daughters were excluded to the line of the person who had actually dowered them; but the exclusion extended to embrace all ascendants and descendants within that line.[103]

Medieval jurists believed that a father was bound not only to dower his daughters but to do so properly—with a dowry whose value was proportionate to his substance. In Italy the statutes of at least one commune, Volterra, required it; and others, like Bologna, demanded at least an equality among daughters.[104] In practice, such ideals were often ignored. Poor Clementia, whose father, William VII of Montpellier, consigned to a nunnery with 20 marks of silver in his will of 1172, had three sisters, each of whom he dowered with 100 marks. That was perhaps a legitimate distinction—the nunnery had a longer life expectancy than a husband and would keep her until her death, whereas her sisters would have to depend in widowhood on their dowries. But even daughters who married were not always treated equally by their fathers. William VIII of Montpellier, in his will of 1202, dowered his daughter Marie with 200 marks and an "honorable trousseau," but his daughters Agnes and Adelaide were to be married with half that amount. Among the Williams of Montpellier, who practised an intricate form of primogeniture which generally made one son heir for life, left one waiting in the wings in case of his death, and made clerics of the rest, daughters, in a sense, received the same treatment as sons.[105] But even in Italy, which seems to have upheld remarkably the principle of equal division among sons, distinctions among daughters, were frequently made. The wills of Genoese fathers usually did award daughters, with the exception of those destined for the convent, dowries of equal value; but we find less equivalence in the actual marriage settlements arranged by living fathers. The dowry at work became divorced from death-bed or legislative ideals. A typical case is that of Orieta Zaccaria, whose dowry of 1000 Genoese pounds (that married her in the mid-thirteenth century to the son of Genoa's ruler) was not matched by those of her sisters or cousins, who took only 600 pounds into their later marriages.[106]

For the humble, a dowry—when it could be scraped up at all—often bore a close relation to a daughter's natural inheritance portion, as it clearly did in the case of a Genoese blacksmith who gave up one-half of his and his wife's estate to marry their daughter in 1190 with a 12 pound dowry.[107] Among wealthier parts of the population, however, the relation was much less firmly established. The record of payment made by the commune of Genoa in 1223 of 3000 Genoese pounds for a portion of the estate of Enrico de Uxecio, a father of four, informs us that he had awarded as dowry to his only daughter a mere 120 pounds, only 70 of which had so far been paid.[108] It gives point to Pope Innocent III's roughly contemporary opinion that the income from dowry was often insufficient to sustain the expenses of a marriage.[109]

A preference for cash dowries throughout the western Mediterranean is a further sign of the daughter's effective disinheritance. A dowry in money was rare in southern France in the eleventh century.[110] But a century later Roger Bernard, Count of Foix, was exceptional among the lords of Languedoc in awarding his daughter a dowry of real property; almost all of his twelfth-century peers offered their daughters cash.[111] And Alphonse II, Count of Provence, stipulated in his will of 1209 that "he wished his daughter Grisenda to be married with money and without [any] part of the land of Provence."[112] In both Montpellier and Barcelona in the thirteenth century dowries frequently contained some real property, but it was generally shaped around a cash base.[113] In Genoa well over 70 percent of the dowries recorded in the city's extant notarial acts were awarded in cash in the thirteenth and fourteenth centuries, as were most in thirteenth-century Siena and in fourteenth- and fifteenth-century Toulouse.[114] Real property was too valuable to be alienated to daughters; and the poor recognized this as clearly as the rich. At Ganges, where dowries were poorer than in neighboring Montpellier, they were more frequently given solely in cash. And real property disappeared from dowries even in Montpellier in the hard times of the late Middle Ages.[115] A similar progress can be detected in Provence, where dowries in real property, which had been prevalent among all but the aristocracy in the fourteenth century, had been transformed into silver by the beginning of the fifteenth.[116]

Within the world of the Italian commune, as undoubtedly elsewhere in aristocratic society, the reluctance to assign real property as dowry was strengthened among the ruling group by their fear that strategic property might thereby fall out of the family; and such property was often made the reserve of the male line. Thus, for example, members of the tower society of Orsanmichele in Florence agreed in 1209 that in the case of the death of one of their number, his share should fall to his sons, grandsons, brothers, or nephews, for "no wife . . . or daughters or sisters or nieces or any other woman should have part or any share in the said tower."[117] A similar sentiment forbade in Salon the dowering in land of daughters who were marrying outside the city.[118] In Barcelona real property may have continued longer to form part of the city's dowries, but it came surprisingly often from a maternal estate and perhaps constituted a separate class of female, dotal property.[119]

Husbands, of course, also preferred cash. Although women retained ownership of the dowry during marriage, their husbands managed it and collected the income. While this management was restricted by the requirement that wives consent to alienation of the dotal fund, a cash dowry could be much more easily merged with the husband's estate. Property in dowry, on the other hand, was a more visible sign of the wife's patrimony. It could be conveyed in either appraised [*estimata*] or unappraised [*inestimata*] goods. The *dos inestimata* preserved more faithfully the regime of separation of goods implicit in the dotal marriage than did the *dos estimata*. The former could not be alienated or exchanged with any ease and would normally be returned intact at the dissolution of the marriage; the latter, whether it consisted of cash or land, was much more easily alienable, since only its assessed worth had to be restored.[120] The striking failure of the *dos inestimata* to establish a secure footing, even in rural areas, may be a sign of the strength of the husband's position.[121]

At the dissolution of her marriage, a woman—provided always that she had not been caught in adultery—could demand from her husband's estate the dowry her father had given her as a bride, which would be her chief support into the grave. In the medieval West this right may have evolved slowly, much as it had in Rome, which had only reluctantly given up the husband's rights of ownership.[122] Some evidence from southern France suggests that initially the dowry awarded in money had been distinguished from a woman's landed inheritance and, unlike that inheritance, had been abandoned to the husband as his real property. Thus Gasinde gave her husband Raymond de Fontjoncoure 1300 solidi in dowry in 1180 or 1182: 650 in cash "to do with as he pleases" and 650 as her "inheritance."[123] But by the thirteenth century the husband was beginning to be obliged to restore an equivalent sum at the dissolution of the marriage.[124] A similar, original distinction between cash and land may also explain why in Barcelona the value of the *escreix* was set in relation to the cash dowry, without regard to the part given in unassessed land.[125] But certainly by the mid-thirteenth century throughout southern Europe a widow's dotal rights had been legally secured. They were not limited by the presence of children; and if they or any of her husband's heirs were slow in repaying her dowry, she was often allowed a living from the estate.[126]

Her predecease was more troublesome. The jurists argued that the dowry should revert not to her husband but either to its donor or to her children (whose father might, however hold it for them).[127] But the husband's privileges were always tenacious. A Barcelonese father made his son-in-law promise in 1221 that if his daughter should die within five years of their marriage, her dowry of 200 solidi must be returned.[128] In a larger sense, the way in which communities wrestled with this central problem of the destination of the dowry in the event of a wife's predecease is a guide to their attitude toward the dotal principle of separation of goods. In some places the counterdower was seen as a guarantee of a husband's share in the dowry should he outlive his wife. Husbands from Genoa and Pavia gained from the dowries of their wives whatever they had contributed as counterdower; where none had been constituted, they received the value of its customary worth—one-half the dowry in Genoa, one-third in Pavia (or 100 pounds in both cities if the dowry was in excess of 200).[129] In other communities strong associative tendencies struggled against dotal demands of separation of goods to maintain for widowers significant rights in the marital estate. The Custom of Montpellier (art. 118) had, for example, assured to husbands usufruct of any real property conveyed as dowry. Of course, the almost total transformation there of dowries into cash in the fourteenth century must have undermined the position of the widowers of Montpellier. Perhaps that is why their wives began at precisely that moment to will them their dowries. Both there and further west, where Roman law had put down more shallow roots and where Visigothic custom encouraged it, examples multiplied in the fourteenth and fifteenth centuries of couples who established communities of goods organized within a dotal regime.[130]

Law and custom were undoubtedly influential in promoting or retarding a full acceptance of dotal principles of separation. Catalonia toyed with community of goods in the thirteenth and fourteenth centuries, to the extent that a "matrimonio mig per mig" established itself as a legal form of marriage in the Custom of Tortosa.[131] But in Barcelona, and indeed throughout Catalonia, where Roman law had established itself fairly early,[132] the dotal regime triumphed.[133] Law and custom could, however, be molded to suit particular economic and social needs. Community managed to flourish in some parts of Italy; and even in Latium, at the very center of Roman tradition, there evolved limited association of goods, which allowed room occasionally for true community.[134]

The case of the artisans of Genoa demonstrates in some detail the influence that social and economic organization could have in defining the nature of the dotal regime. Like the patriciate that ruled the city, Genoa's artisan community—always poor and insignificant by Florentine standards—dowered its daughters and gave counterdowers (*antefactum*) to its wives; and along with aristocratic women, the city's artisan wives had lost their right to *tercia* in 1143. But unlike patricians, artisans steadfastly refused to yield to the spirit of that law which had also set a limit (of one-half the dowry or 100 Genoese pounds, whichever was the lesser sum) on *antefactum*. Although in fewer than half of the extant patrician marriage contracts of the twelfth century did women receive a settlement from their husbands that was in excess of the prescribed limit, in over seventy percent of artisan contracts, *antefactum* exceeded half the dowry's value. Moreover, the contrast grew in the following centuries as patrician dowries climbed to 1000, even 2000 Genoese pounds—while artisan dowries often failed to exceed 100. As patrician husbands of the fourteenth and fifteenth centuries regularly awarded their wives the prescribed *antefactum* of 100 pounds, artisans continued to flout the law and often awarded counterdowers that equalled the value of the dowry they had received.[135] Thus while patrician widows and widowers had no more than a small, symbolic claim on the other's estate, artisans, on the death of a spouse, frequently gained control of the whole conjugal fund. In Genoa the patriciate adopted dotal separation, but its artisans opted for community.

Generally, however, the introduction of the dotal regime into Mediterranean marriage drew attention away from the conjugal bond to focus it instead on the relations between the couple and the wife's kinsmen, whose rights toward children of the marriage dowry guaranteed. In Siena, for instance, the presence of a dowry allowed the wife's family formally to participate in the upbringing of her children.[136] Their right to step in if the husband mismanaged the dotal fund may, furthermore, have promoted that association between brothers-in-law that is characteristic of business life within the patriciates of some late medieval cities—an association in which the wife's brother almost invariably assumed the dominant role.[137] Within a woman's own family, dowry must inevitably have centered attention on the father-daughter bond; for daughters would live all their lives in the light of their father's generosity or in the shadow of its absence. Gratian (in his influential *Decretum* of about 1140) had given support to the view that the consent of marital partners was necessary for a true marriage—at precisely that time when the net of dotal marriage was catching daughters ever more firmly in the marital schemes of their kinsmen. If his final position would probably not have gone as far as his rubric "A father's oath cannot force a girl to marry one to whom she has never assented," such a belief did form part of Peter Lombard's radical theory of consent that less than twenty years later began to push the Church toward the essentially consensual definition of marriage that it would retain until the Council of Trent.[138] But it was never fully embraced by the dotal world, where customary and statute law often deprived of dowry any woman who married against her father's will.[139]

Her father and her dowry became the chief protectors and guarantors of a girl's sexual purity. And society recognized in the undowered woman a threat to its moral stability. The Genoese chronicler Giorgio Stella claimed that the ruin of patrician fortunes at the beginning of the fourteenth century, by depriving girls of their dowries and thus delaying marriages within the city, had forced many women to "stain their bodily honor in venal commerce, driven by poverty, that teacher of corruption[140]—perhaps rather like those Lydian prostitutes Herodotus noticed (I.93), who converted their profits into dowries. Such considerations undoubtedly lay behind the dowering of poor girls as an increasingly popular form of private and public charity and the insistence of governmental leaders and ecclesiastical authorities on a father's obligation to dower his daughters. The petition to King Joan I in 1390 by Eulàlia, the daughter of a Barcelonese notary whose refusal to dower her had left the woman unmarried into her late twenties, brought the decision that her father must supply her with a fitting dowry,[141] a decision that both the governments of the Italian communes and jurists would have defended. Pope Benedict XII viewed as sufficient grounds for allowing the marriage, contracted within the forbidden degree of consanguinity, between the Genoese patrician Tropa Cattaneo and his poor, but aristocratic bride Salvagia Lercari the fact that the groom had constituted his wife's dowry. This obviously shameful defect was better kept within the family.[142] Generally, however, fathers committed themselves to giving chaste, dowered daughters into marriage. The growing association between dowry and chastity may be one reason why aristocratic Italian fathers—unlike Lombard ones, who had allowed their daughters to grow old at home[143]—so often married their daughters off at puberty.[144] A father's concern for the sexual behavior of his daughter continued, however, beyond her marriage; for the adulterous woman lost to her husband the dowry that might otherwise (in the absence of children) have reverted to her own kin. In the dotal world of the Mediterranean, there was an economics of shame.

IV

The extensiveness of marriage gifts lends both strength and instability to the systems of which they form a part. As signs of the bundle of rights and obligations that their giving and receipt impose down a long chain on both sides of the marital divide, they bind those who have exchanged them into a new community which thereby has vested interests in the marriage. The wide variety of gifts and countergifts, givers and receivers, means that any one system of marital assigns contains aspects of the others. Our definition of a particular system really describes a point of balance. And we must now briefly face the question of why that point shifts, as it did at least twice in the European Middle Ages, as it probably did in the ancient world, and as it does within some societies today.

If we isolate the marital couple from the larger system, the exchange of marital assigns can assume the aspect of a marketplace; and laws of supply and demand might seem a way of explaining change: men paid for brides in the early Middle Ages because brides were so scarce, their numbers depleted by the trials of childbearing in so primitive and warlike a society. In those parts of Albania where men recently paid brideprice, it was put proverbially: "A woman's grave is always open."[145] Women paid dowry in the later period, so the argument runs, because marriageable men had become scarcer, their numbers reduced so by the practice of primogeniture in some places, collective restraint in others, that, in the words of Alain de Lille, "The natural anvils bewail the absence of their hammers and are seen sadly to demand them."[146]

This is not a new argument. It has been used to explain the rise in the value of dowries in ancient Sparta and the change from *hedna* to dowry marriage throughout the Greek world.[147] But apart from the unreliability of the demographic evidence on which we must rely in the early medieval period,[148] there is some positive evidence against such an easy interpretation of change. In a situation of early medieval scarcity, one might expect women to improve their status through advantageous marriage. Why then were Lombard women being kept at home so long that—in what must have been desperation—they married into the slave class, an offense for which the punishment was servitude and possibly even death?[149] Nor does such a demographic hypothesis explain either the devaluation of brideprice throughout the Germanic world or the steady increase in value, in both Visigothic Spain and Lombard Italy, in the gifts that husbands awarded at marriage to their wives. Unless one posits a sudden shift in the sex ratio or in marital practices—a shift for which no evidence has been advanced—demography cannot tell us why a supposedly perennial shortage of women would suddenly provoke change.[150]

Questions of supply and demand might seem to be more pertinent in the later period, from about the eleventh century. The remarkably well-documented case of the upwardly mobile Vivas family of Barcelona, for example, suggests that its success lay in a familial coherence based on a policy that allowed only one son to marry. Yet, as the 1053 will of Pere Vivas shows, more daughters were expected to enjoy the wedded state; and Pere was willing to pay out for the dowries of his two daughters over 65 ounces of gold, a sum that could buy six or seven war horses or a couple of fortresses and which was more than he had ever expended in his career.[151] The wills of the lords of Montpellier also show that at the very moment that the old marital assigns were dying in Languedoc more sons than daughters were being forced into celibacy and away from the marriage market.[152] It might seem tempting to suggest that principles of primogeniture among the landed classes combined with strategies of delayed marriage within some urban patriciates to produce an excess of marriageable women, who were then forced to bear dowries into marriage.[153] Yet the fairly consistent taste of widowers for young, virgin brides and the frequent reluctance of aristocratic widows to remarry might have served to balance the sex ratio of the marriageable. Unless more telling demographic evidence can be advanced, an argument based on supply and demand must remain a weak one.

A link with inheritance practices seems more important. When we place the rise in *morgengabe* in the context of a system of assigns that may continue throughout the marriage and into the next generation, we notice that its most striking feature is the concentration of assigns around the conjugal pair and the children of the match—away from the larger kin group. The rise in *morgengabe* coincided precisely among the Lombards, for example, with growing recognition of the inheritance rights of daughters at the expense of the non-lineal kin group[154]—a group that was also deprived of its unchallenged control over the estates of fatherless children by King Aistulf's concession to the popular demand that widows might be given usufruct of their husbands' estates.[155] In other words, in both its symbolic and economic support of the conjugal bond, *morgengabe* and the system of assigns of which it formed a part championed the conjugal family, which some evidence is beginning to suggest formed a basic social cell of southern Europe in the Carolingian Age.[156]

In the same light, the so-called rise of dowry might be seen as a sorting out of rights, which were returned to the newly strengthened kin groups that would dominate both city and countryside in the High Middle Ages.[157] Renewed lineal organization had begun to weaken the authority of the conjugal bond. The unwillingness of husbands (and their kin) to assign important parts of their patrimony to wives is one sign of a kin group restrengthened on patrilineal principles, and the securing of a daughter's inheritance in a dowry that gave her rights and status in her husband's home, gained her kinsmen rights in her offspring, and deprived her of substantial landed wealth from her natal patrimony shows the other side of similar patrilineal concerns. Perhaps men now preferred to endow the female members of their own descent group to their wives, who were necessarily alien members since both custom and ecclesiastical law required exogamy.[158] Perhaps too, dowry served as a bridge between these increasingly strong kin solidarities—a mechanism for alliance in an age that was searching for new ways to forge social, economic, and political bonds.

These were necessary in a world where demographic growth, land shortage, and unprecedented commercial development were creating in both cities and countryside a crisis of status. Dowry had been linked to status from the beginning of its renewed association with the marriage contract. When, for example, in his will of 1154, Raymond Trencavel, Viscount of Beziers, made his son heir and dowered his two daughters, he arranged that the younger should marry William of Montpellier with a dowry of 20,000 solidi—if he would have her. If she was rejected, however, she was to receive only half that amount.[159] With this dowry Raymond sought to buy his son an alliance that would increase his status within the southwestern aristocracy. But the other side of the arrangement was that his daughter's status came to be defined by the dowry she bore. With 20,000 solidi she might be mistress of Montpellier; at half that amount her social position would be significantly reduced. Nowhere was this clearer than in the more mobile world of the Renaissance Italian city, which actually came to define a woman's status for some legal purposes according to the value of her dowry. Genoa's fifteenth-century sumptuary laws drew the distinction very carefully, aligning the richness of dress allowed to a woman with the amount of her dowry.[160] If they were obeyed, a well-dowered Genoese woman would have been immediately recognizable by the clothes that the city allowed her to wear.

It was its use as a mechanism for alliance and mobility in a status-conscious yet mobile world that may have encouraged the dowry to rise dramatically in value in the late Middle Ages and in the Renaissance. Dante's lament for a finer age when

> A daughter's birth did not yet fill
> A father's heart with fear,
> For age and dowry had not yet fled to opposite
> extremes (Paradiso, XV: 103-5)[161]

seems to have touched on real social change. Initially, as we have seen, dowries had about them the scent of *disinheritance,* consolation for an exclusion from succession that was increasingly secured in Mediterranean Europe by entail fortified by female renunciations.[162] Yet where wealth and status were not balanced the dowry often came to secure for some daughters a larger slice of the patrimony. Nowhere was this clearer than in the Italian commune. In Savona, for instance, patrician dowries had risen strikingly in the first two decades of the thirteenth century as families with new fortunes used the dowry as a mechanism for alliance and the acquisition of status.[163] Men like Pietro Allichini, the son of a taverner who had become a judge in Padua and who—before he was torn to pieces by a Paduan mob in 1314 for his usury and extortion—married his daughter into a great Paduan family with an extravagant dowry of 3000 pounds, saw their own status reflected in their daughters' dowries.[164] The economic crisis of the later Middle Ages may, moreover, have pushed dowry further along the road toward full inheritance for at least some daughters; the dowered daughter was a symbol of status in an environment where symbols had become ever more important as fortunes seemed ephemeral and status ill-defined. Dowry negotiations were followed avidly by the citizens of Renaissance Italy, who understood their every nuance. For each Florentine who might worry, as one did, that the false rumor that he had dowered his daughter with 2000 florins might ruin his tax position,[165] there were many more who sought to hide the reduced dowries that their daughters carried into marriage, which might deprive the family of community status, even perhaps of a favorable credit rating. Such concerns may have prompted the contributions made to dowries by paternal kinswomen in Renaissance Venice and elsewhere in Italy,[166] but the association between dowry and familial status largely accentuated the interdependence of fathers and their daughters. It may eventually have encouraged the full integration of daughters into the lineage, evidence of which can be found everywhere in southern Europe by the fifteenth and sixteenth centuries in the preference of daughters over collateral males in matters of inheritance.[167]

The fullest rights may have been reserved for those daughters who managed to combine devotion to the lineal and conjugal bond through uxorilocal marriage. For petty agriculturalists, such marriage frequently encouraged an "affrèrement entre époux" in which, in a sense, the man joined his wife's domestic group as both husband and brother.[168] At the more elevated level of the aristocracy, it could mean the incorporation of a man into the lineage of his heiress-wife. Giovanni Grimaldi, who ruled Monaco in the fifteenth century, provided in his will, for example, that should his only son die without a male heir, the estate was to descend to his son's daughter on the condition that she marry a member of the *albergo* Grimaldi,[169] a condition extended in the wills of later rulers to allow husbands who would enter the *albergo* and take the name Grimaldi.[170] But the formula may have been devised by the Grimaldi for use in Genoa some years earlier: when Niccola Grimaldi was faced with the fact of five daughters and no son, he married four outside the *albergo;* to the fifth, Violantina, he assigned enlarged inheritance rights and a husband who entered the *albergo* Grimaldi.[171]

The presence of heiresses, of course, further encouraged dotal inflation, which was—in the eyes of fathers—the curse of early modern Europe. "Vanity of vanities," cried Charles Grimaldi, president of the parlement of Aix in the early seventeenth century, and distant descendant of Grimaldi from Genoa who had experienced the phenomenon centuries earlier, "all is vanity. We kill ourselves, we're numbed and rattled by settling a daughter and making a good alliance; but we don't always succeed. . . . It is not prudent to damage a house for the dowry of daughters."[172] But, of course, many did; for the status of the house seemed often to hang on it. In some places, demographic factors may have contributed to the dotal inflation endemic in early modern Europe, as in England where primogeniture, hypergamy, and the abolition of religious houses seem to have combined to supply ever more women and fewer men for the aristocratic marriage market.[173] But we should remember that the cities of Italy, which did not practise primogeniture,[174] which upheld chastity as a feminine ideal, and which maintained the nunnery as a "convenient stowage for their withered daughters" had experienced dotal inflation as soon as dowry became associated with an active marriage policy. If in Renaissance Italy, as in early modern England, the reluctance of fathers to marry their daughters down and their willingness to accept large dowries from wives of lesser status for their sons contributed to dotal inflation, such hypergamy is a sign of the powerful links that had been forged between daughters, dowries, and family status.

The medieval Mediterranean dowry—like those in Ceylon and other parts of Asia[175]—almost from its beginnings, then, formed part of a status, rather than an inheritance system. Only where status concerns were minimal—as, for instance, among Genoa's petty artisans—did dowry resemble natural inheritance; and there, since it was part of a balanced marriage settlement in which the husband's contribution remained so important, it is probably misleading to speak of "dotal marriage." Dowry flourished to drive out other marital assigns where men used their rights over the women of their lineage, particularly their daughters, as a way of asserting status or competing for it. Far from being a daughter's simple or natural inheritance claim in a system of bilateral descent, as Goody has suggested, the medieval Mediterranean dowry rose to prominence as a form of disinheritance within a social group whose organization had become significantly *less* bilateral. Perhaps, ironically, only the increased status that daughters derived from the heightened dowries of the later Middle Ages eventually won them more extensive inheritance rights in their patrilineage.

It was *morgengabe* and its associated portion—the husband's gift to his bride—that seems, from beginning to end, to have been most closely associated with bilateral descent. The Lombards, for example, had begun to reject the principles of unilineal descent at precisely the moment that *morgengabe* began its rise at the expense of bridewealth. And it was the aristocracy's turning from bilateral principles that everywhere drove this assign into oblivion. Yet the husband's gift to his wife flourished in Mediterranean Europe for almost five centuries; and it may have left its mark even upon the aristocracy, who were first to reject it, in the continued concern that husbands expressed in the sexual conduct of their wives. In some places the association between the husband's gift and virginity remained strong even after its real value had begun to decline. In Amalfi "quarta" was awarded to a wife "only by that husband who deflowered [*corrupit*] her";[176] and in Catalonia some wedding charters continued to award the *escreix* (a gift tied closely to the dowry) "in recognition of virginity" into the sixteenth century.[177] Adulterous women of all social groups were subject to extreme punishment—death in some parts of Italy and Spain, a humiliatingly public and naked race elsewhere.[178] Toward the end of the Middle Ages and in the Renaissance, however, especially where dowry had made its most striking gains, the sexual power of husbands over wives may have declined—introducing into Mediterranean society the *cicisbeo,* or gallant, and popularizing in its literature the cuckold. It is a process visible along the northern Mediterranean littoral as early as the twelfth century in the poetry of the troubadours, whose rise was contemporary with the decline of the husband's gift.

We should like to know what effects such changes had among the parts of the population that did not wholeheartedly embrace "dotal marriage" and whether similar ambiguities in the husband's position can be found in other dotal areas, both those of ancient times and those which practise dowry marriage today. They are important questions; for in the history of the competition, both material and psychological, between the husband's gift, and the bilateral and conjugal principles on which it rested, and the dowry, the symbol of patrilineal status, may lie a deeply original contribution of the medieval world to the larger development of Mediterranean culture and society.

REFERENCES

1. *Iliad* 22:472. Aristotle, *The Politics.* Translated by Ernest Barker (New York and London, 1958) 2:viii 1268 b 39. *Hedna* is an almost exclusively Homeric word used, usually in the plural, to signify wedding gifts. It has been proposed that it derives from Indo-European **wed-no-*; and a relation has been seen with the Old Russian *veno,* meaning brideprice or husband's gift. (Pierre Chantraine, *Dictionnaire étymologique de la langue grecque* [Paris, 1968] 2:312).

2. M. Moritz Voigt, *Die XII Tabeln.* 2 vols. (Leipzig, 1883) 2:704.

3. Walter Erdmann, *Die Ehe im alten Griechenland* (Munich, 1934), 218-20; Hans Julius Wolff, "Die Grundlagen des griechischen Eherechte," *Tijdschrift voor Rechtsgeschiedenis* 20 (1952): 1-29; 157-81; *Odyssey* 1:275-78; *Iliad* 9:146-57. The expression by which he designates this gift is *meilia,* the Greek form of the Church Slavic *milo,* meaning dowry (H. d'Arbois de Jubainville, *La famille celtique* [Osnabrück, 1970, reprint], 60), but not the term used to signify that gift in the classical period.˙

4. R. Köstler, "Raub-, Kauf- und Friedelehe bei den Germanen," *Zeitschrift der Savigny-Stiftung für Rechtsgeschichte,* Germ Abt. 63 (1943): 92-136.

5. M.I. Finley, "Marriage, Sale and Gift in the Homeric World," *Revue internationale des droits de l'antiquité,* 3d ser., 2(1955): 194. P. Koschaker, "Eheformen bei den Indogermanen," *Zeitschrift fur Auslandisches und Internationales Privatrecht* 11 (1937): 77-140.

6. Hans Julius Wolff, "Marriage Law and Family Organization in Ancient Athens," *Traditio* 2 (1944): 44-46.

7. Edoardo Volterra, "La conception du mariage à Rome," *Revue internationale des droits de l'antiquité,* 3d ser., 2 (1955): 366.

8. 2:vv. 689-91. Plautus, of course, was heavily influenced by Greek literary example.

9. d'Arbois de Jubainville, *La famille celtique,* 113-24; Louis M. Epstein, *The Jewish Marriage Contract* (New York, 1973, reprint), 53-77; A.S. Diamond, *Primitive Law Past and Present* (London, 1971), 82-103.

10. Samuel Greengus, "Old Babylonian Marriage Ceremonies and Rites," *Journal of Cuneiform Studies* 20 (1966): 57-72; "The Old Babylon Marriage Contract," *Journal of the American Oriental Society* 89 (1969): 505-32. C.H.N. Johns, *Babylonian and Assyrian Laws, Contracts and Letters* (Edinburgh, 1904), 71, 125-26. These later records use for dowry not the term *seriktu,* but *nudunnu,* which appears in the Code of Hammurabi as a husband's gift to his bride, a transferral of meaning that may resemble that contained in Penelope's *hedna.*

11. P.W. Pestman, *Marriage and Matrimonial Property in Ancient Egypt* (Leiden, 1961), 6-52.

12. Fourteen percent of Circum-Mediterranean societies, nine percent of East Eurasian, practice dotal marriage. This is merely a rough figure, for the categories need to be redefined. Goody has pointed out that one of its most misleading features is the classification of the husband's gift to the bride under the category of bridewealth (Jack R. Goody and S.J. Tambiah, *Bridewealth and Dowry* [Cambridge, 1973], 21-22).

13. *Joshua* 15:18-19; *Judges* 1:15; *Tobias* 8:24; Epstein, *The Jewish Marriage Contract,* 53-77. One Indo-European exception seems to have been the Armenians (d'Arbois de Jubainville, *La famille celtique,* 59).

14. Goody and Tambiah, *Bridewealth and Dowry,* 1-2, 22-23.

15. Strabo, *The Geography,* trans. Horace Leonard Jones. 8 vols. (London and New York, 1917-1949) 2: 15. G. Paturet, *De la condition juridique de la femme dans l'ancienne Egypte* (Paris, 1886), 51.

16. The Greek dotal system did incorporate a more generous contribution from the husband, a return gift for the dowry, which eventually made headway in Rome in the late Empire (Lucien Anné, *Les rites des fiançailles et la donation pour cause de mariage sous le Bas-Empire* [Louvain, 1941]); but Rome's dependence on either Greek or Eastern institutions in its development of the husband's donation or the betrothal guarantee (through *arra sponsalicia*) is probably further testimony to the early dominance of dotal marriage in Rome.

17. The Roman Empire exercised authority over many peoples who, like the Celts, continued to know marriage with brideprice (although Celtic women also received dowries from their own kinsmen [Caesar 6:18.1]); and this may have made them receptive to the Germanic system of marital assigns.

18. André Lemaire believed that Leo's letter referred to similar earlier legislation by Theodosius ("Nullum sine dote fiat conjugium," in *Mélanges Paul Fournier* [Paris, 1929], 414-24); but there is no certain evidence to support one side or the other. His letter of 458 could not, of course, inform the West that the Constitution (if it is indeed this to which he referred) would be rescinded in 463, a fact of which even Gratian seems to have been unaware (Decretum, C.30 q.55c.3, in Emil Friedberg, ed., *Corpus Juris Canonici* [Graz, 1955, reprint],1). The requirement became enshrined in some Germanic legal codes. Among the Visigoths, the association of the husband's donation with a legal marriage was first made by King Ervig (Karolus Zeumer, ed., *Leges Visigothorum,* Monumenta Germaniae Historica [hereafter MGH], Legum Sectio I, i [Hanover, 1902] III.19), but P.D. King is right to challenge Lemaire's assertion that marriage without it was henceforth considered invalid (King, *Law and Society in the Visigothic Kingdom* [Cambridge, 1972], 225-26). The Burgundian Code, however, did make the validity of a marriage dependent on the presence of the husband's gift (*donatio nuptialis*) even among the Roman population (L.R. de Salis, ed., *Leges Burgundionum* MGH, Legum Sectio I, ii (1) [Hanover, 1892], XXXVII, 1.; Heinrich Brunner, *Abhandlungen zur Rechtsgeschichte* [Leipzig, 1965] 1:90-92). For Nicholas' influential letter, see Epistolae Nicolae I papae, 99, in E. Perls, ed., *Epistolae Karolini Aevi* IV, MGH [Berlin, 1925], 569-70.

19. In Montpellier, for example, the same long, formulaic preamble that a generation

earlier had introduced the conveyal of the husband's gift was in the twelfth century being used to open dotal charters (Jean Hilaire, *Le régime des biens entre époux dans la région de Montpellier du debut du XIIIe siècle à la fin du XVIe siècle* [Montpellier, 1957], introduction). And when in Florence Dante and Villani looked back to the good old days before extravagant dowries had begun to ruin the virtue of the city and its women, neither looked beyond, into the time of the husband's gift (*La Divina Commedia, Paradiso* 15:103-5; G. Villani, *Cronica* [Florence, 1823], 2:96).

20. Quoted by Nino Tamassia, *La famiglia italiana nei secoli decimoquinto e decimosesto* (Rome, 1971, reprint), 301, n.1.

21. Elizabeth Rawson, *The Spartan Tradition in European Thought* (Oxford, 1969), 136.

22. Since the formality of legal codes tends to conceal diversity of practice, which we cannot usually recover in the absence of charters, the clarity or uniformity of practice in the earliest period may be more apparent than real. Furthermore, the timelessness of both the Germanic codes and later customals poses another problem. Customs drawn from an undifferentiated past can mislead concerning the social behavior of the present, which it may or may not wholly or in part reflect (Diane O. Hughes, "Toward Historical Ethnography: Notarial Records and Family History in the Middle Ages," *Historical Methods Newsletter* 7:51-71). In the case of customals, however, we are often able to gain precision through the use of charter and urban statutes. And although the codes will always be difficult, those issued by the tribes that settled along the northern shore of the Mediterranean are usually more chronologically precise than those of other tribes.

23. Marcel Mauss, *The Gift*, tr. Ian Cannson (London, 1954). Its obligatory nature is fairly fully defined in the Lombard Code, where it is called *laungild* (*Leges Langobardorum*, Franz Beyerle, ed., 2d ed. [Witzenhausen, 1962], Edictum Rotharii 175, 184; Liutprand 43.XIV, 54.I, 73.IV; Aistulf, 12.III).

24. *Germania*. J.G.C. Anderson, ed., *Cornelii Taciti Opera Minora* (Oxford, 1958), 18.

25. Norden established, of course, that Tacitus had taken much from Pliny's lost *Bella Germaniae;* but it is worth noting that the contents of the husband's donation that he describes resemble quite strikingly those described in the only full Germanic lists we have, lists for *morgengabe* among the Visigoths. Cornuey, in his otherwise helpful study of the husband's gift (L.M.A. Cornuey, *Le régime de la "dos" aux époques merovingienne et carolingienne* [Algiers, 1929]), argued without any substantial evidence to support his case that the gift described was brideprice.

26. Fredegarius, *Cronica*, ed. B. Krusch (MGH, 1889, *Scriptorum rerum merovingicarum*) 2:III.18; K. Zeumer, *Formulae merowingici et karolini aevi* (Hanover, 1882-1886), MGH, Legum sectio V., 230, 247-48, 271; A. Vandenbossche, *La "dos ex marito" dans la Gaule franque* (Paris, 1953), pt. 2; Leges Saxonum, MGH, Legum Sectio v (Hanover, 1875-1889), 43, 49. I am not arguing here for "marriage by purchase," which Köstler ("Raub-, Kauf- und Friedelehe") has denied for Germanic as for Greco-Roman society and which is an anachronism in any case in a society whose economy is characterized by exchange rather than sale. Yet the equation, both in Saxon and Lombard legislation, of the value of *wergeld* and brideprice does seem to suggest that the brideprice was exchanged in a fairly direct way for judicial rights over the woman.

27. *Leges Burgundionum*, Gundobad 66, 86. Elsewhere in the Code, *wittimon* is translated as *pretium nuptiale* (12.4; 52.3), *pretium uxoris* (54.3), and *pretium puellae* (12.2). *Leges Visigothorum*, III:1.2, III:2.8, III:3.3, III:4.2, III:4.7; Paulo Merêa, *Estudios de direito visigotico* (Coimbra, 1948).

28. Linguistic evidence actually points to West German origins for them; but their institutions were much closer to the Scandinavian Germans. Perhaps their long sojourn among ancestors of the Saxons shaped them in ways unknown to us (Lucien Musset, *Les invasions: les vagues germaniques* [Paris, 1969], 138-39).

29. *Leges Langobardorum*, Edictum Rotharii, Art. 178; Liutprand 89, vi. Art. 178 of Rothair's edict seems to suggest that only in the case of a broken betrothal did a woman re-

ceive *meta,* as a kind of compensation; but the wording is ambiguous, and it may be that even in Rothair's day women regularly received their *meta.*

30. F. Brandileone, *Scritti di storia del diritto privato italiano* (Bologna, 1931), 229-319.

31. Under Visigothic law, the possessor of the *potestas de coniunctione* had almost complete control over a girl's marriage until she reached the age of twenty. Although any marriage she might contract without the consent of that guardian was regarded as valid, she forfeited all rights in her paternal and maternal inheritance. After the age of twenty, however, she seems to have become entirely free to contract her own marriage, both as a spinster and as a widow (P.D. King, *Law and Society in the Visigothic Kingdom* [Cambridge, 1972], 225-6). Among both the Visigoths and the Burgundians (R. de Hubé, "Histoire de la formation de loi bourguignonne," *Revue historique de droit français et étranger* 13 [1867]:209-59), the concept of *mundium* was losing its force.

32. Pietro Vaccari, *Scritti di storia del diritto privato* (Padua, 1966), 7-8; A. Lemaire, "La dotatio de l'épouse de l'époque mérovingienne au XIIIe siècle," *Revue historique de droit français et étranger* 4th ser., 8(1929): 569-88. It has been proposed that the Germans, like other Indo-European peoples, had always known a variety of forms of marriage, one of which left the woman her husband's equal partner, not subject to his legal authority. Meyer has drawn attention, for example, to the popular practice (which he feels faithfully reflects primitive German custom) of *Friedelverhältniss.* He describes this not as concubinage but as a marriage of equals in which the woman's *mundium* was never rewarded in return for brideprice. Instead, she was recognized as a wife by her husband's award of *morgengabe* (Herbert Meyer, "Friedelehe und Mutterrecht," *Zeitschrift der Savigny-Stiftung für Rechtsgeschichte,* Germ. Abt. 47[1927]:198-226). For Meyer, marriage with *mundium* was patriarchal marriage; *Friedelehe* represented an earlier matriarchal institution. But this theory has been generally attacked: see Simon Kalifa, "Singularités matrimoniales chez les anciens germains: le rapt et le droit de la femme à disposer d'elle-même," *Revue historique de droit français et étranger* 4th ser., 48(1970): 199-225, with extensive bibliographic reference.

33. Gregory of Tours, *The History of the Franks,* trans. O.M. Dalton, 2 vols. (Oxford, 1927), 9:20; *Lex Ribuaria,* Franz Beyerle and Rudolph Buchner, eds. MGH, Legum Sectio I, iii(2) (Hanover, 1954), XLVI:11. A morning gift representing one-quarter of the *wergeld* of a freeman may well have been devised under the influence of Justinian's Novella 22 (ch. 18), which allowed to poor widows one-quarter of their husband's substance (Juliette M. Turlan, "Recherches sur la quarte du conjoint pauvre," *Revue historique de droit français et étranger* 4th ser., 44[1966]: 210-39).

34. *Leges Burgondionum,* Gundobad, 24. If she had children, a widow received usufruct of the *donatio* while she lived; and at her death it was divided among her children or their heirs. If the marriage had produced no children, her kinsmen received half of the *donatio* on her death and her husband's kinsmen the other half.

35. Nibelungenlied, 19. *The Fall of the Nibelungs,* trans. Margaret Armour (London, 1897).

36. *Leges Visigothorum,* III:1.5; Zeumer, *Formulae merowingici et karolini aevi,* 584.

37. Luigi Schiaparelli, ed., *Codice diplomatico Langobardo* (Rome, 1929) 1:68. A charter dated from the previous year, also from Lucca, records the donation by the nun Astrualda, acting with the consent of her son, of a house and lands that formed part of her *morgengabe* (ibid., 67).

38. Zeumer, *Formulae merowingici et karolini aevi,* 584.

39. This would seem to be the sense of Chindasvind's legislation, which mentions the 1000 solidi and slaves and horses at the beginning of the law in connection with the rights of *primates palatii;* he concludes, in a way that seems to embrace all free Visigoths, to allow "ut qui in rebus omnibus decem milium solidorum dominus esse dinoscitur, ad mille solidos, rerum universarum contropatione havita, in nomine isponse sue dotem conscribat. Cui autem mille solidorum facultas est, de centum solidis tali aderatione dotem facturus est." Ervig's law makes a clear distinction between the 1000 solidi and the additional grant of one-tenth;

but he may have intended the 1000 solidi as a ceiling on slaves, horses, and ornaments; see A. Schultze, *Über westgotisch-spanisches Eherecht* (Leipzig, 1943), 44-54. Although the influence of Roman practices and legislation on the development of the Germanic husband's gift was clearly significant (Brunner, *Abhandlungen zur Rechtsgeschichte*), Otero is clearly wrong to equate the Visigothic *dos* exclusively with the roman *donatio ante nuptias* and to deny the presence of *morgengabe.*

40. Antonio C. Floriano, ed., *Diplomatico espanola del periodo astur,* 2 vols. (Oviedo, 1949-1951), 2: doc. 139.

41. *Leges Langobardorum,* Liutprand 7.I.

42. *Leges Burgundionum,* Gundobad 42. A widow with children was similarly to receive usufruct of one-third of her husband's property (ibid, 62).

43. *Lex Ribuaria* 41, i, ii.

44. Vandenbossche, *La "dos ex marito,"* part 1.

45. But this may have been common practice much earlier. Fredegar (*Cronica* 4:85) relates that at the death of King Dagobert in 639, his queen received one-third of what he had acquired (Brunner, *Abhandlungen zur Rechtsgeschichte,* 114).

46. Lemaire, "Les origines de la communauté de biens entre époux dans le droit coutumier français," *Revue historique de droit français et étranger* 4th ser., 7 (1928): 584-643.

47. *Leges Alamannorum,* Karolus Lehmann, ed., MGH, Legum Sectio, I, vi (1) (Hanover, 1888), E Codd A LIV, 3.

48. According to the provisions in the Alamannic Code, a childless widow who wished to leave her former husband's estate to marry was to receive, in addition to her own goods, *dotis legitima.* Its value varies greatly—from 40 to 400 solidi—among the different manuscript copies of the Code. If her husband's kinsmen contested her right to this grant and if she reclaimed it by oath or battle, it fell totally into her power and reverted at her death to her next husband or to their children. Though she could certainly claim on her husband's death whatever *morgengabe* he had awarded her, the law does not specify its recipient in the event of her death.

49. *Leges Burgundionum,* Gundobad, 24. *Leges Visigothorum,* IV.2.14. This law probably shows the influence of Justinian's Novella 117, ch. 5, which provided that if a man had at least three children, his widow received usufruct rights in the estate equal to the share of one child; but this legislation of Justinian, rather surprisingly, remained little known and used in southern France until the sixteenth century (Turlan, "Recherches sur la quarte.").

50. *Nibelungenlied,* 19.

51. In Catalonia a similar division into a specific grant of "sponsalitium" and the more generalized tenth (Barcelona, Archivo Capitular Div. B 913, 1783) may have had similar origins, as perhaps did the separate grants of *tercia* and *antefactum* in Liguria, although Brandileone, citing the example of a woman living by Roman law who disposed of her *antefactum* and *morgengabe* in 1095 (*Scritti di storia,* 278), has suggested that *antefactum* had its origin in the Roman counterdower, which continued to be given long after the dowry had lost its earlier significance.

52. A. Bernard and A. Bruel, eds., *Recueil des chartes de l'abbaye de Cluny* (Paris, 1876-1903), 1: docs. 189-90. In the Burgundian documents the grant is called either *sponsalitium* or *dotalitium.* Some historians have maintained a rigorous difference between the two, suggesting either that *sponsalitium* was a prenuptial gift in determined goods while *dotalitium* was given before or after the marriage as a fraction of an estate or of the fruits of the marriage, or that *dotalitium* was a Germanic assign, *sponsalitium* a Roman one. There is evidence for both views; but the charter of 968/9 by which a man awarded his wife goods "in dotalicio et in esponcalitium" (Cluny 2: doc. 1242) suggests that the two often merged.

53. Ibid., doc. 105; Brandileone, *Scritta di storia,* 304-5.

54. P. Merêa, *Estudos de direito hispanico medieval,* 3 vols. (Coimbra, 1952), 1: docs. 69-77; David Herlihy, "*Land, Family and Women in Continental Europe,* 701-1200," *Traditio* 18 (1962). Herlihy's failure to distinguish between single, married, and widowed women makes his statistical study of early charter evidence hard to use with precision.

Toubert has pointed out the important differences between single and married women (Pierre Toubert, *Les structures du Latium médiéval,* 2 vols. [Rome, 1973], 1:766-67); so too the position of a married woman and widow differed significantly, and the status of the latter was clearly colored by the presence or absence of children. Only a study that uses painstaking prosoprographical methods can attain the precision necessary to allow significant comparisons.

55. Cluny 1: docs. 7, 516.

56. Armando Petrucci, ed., *Codice diplomatico del monastero benedettino di S. Maria di Tremiti* (Rome, 1960), nos. 41, 51; Franco Ercole, "Vincende storiche della romana nella pratica medievale dell'Italia superiore," *Archivio giuridico* 80 (1908), 37-38, nn. 3-5, 7-8.

57. Burgues, *Les garanties de restitution de la dot en Languedoc, des invasions barbares â la fin de l'Ancien Rêgime* (Paris, 1937), ch. 1. For Burgundy I have used the charters of Cluny; for Italy the many volumes of charters edited in the *Regesta Chartarum Italiae.*

58. Gregory of Tours, *History of the Franks,* VI, 45.

59. *Leges Visigothorum,* III:1.5; *Leges Langobardorum,* Edictum Rotharii, 181; Liutprand, 102.VII. This would be the case if a father left a son and a daughter; if there were two sons, the daughter (or daughters) received a seventh, and so on.

60. Strictly speaking, of course, it was not until late imperial times that the dowry became necessary for a valid marriage in Rome.

61. That this late, garbled account contains substantial truth is suggested by Aistulf's first law by which he revoked all gifts made by King Ratchis and his wife Tassia. Toubert suggests that the mention of *donationes cartulae romanae* (in the plural) is evidence of the continued existence of the dotal system of Justinian among the Roman population of that area (*Les structures du Latium médiêval,* 1:751-52, n.3).

62. Antonio Marongiû, *La famiglia nell'Italia meridionale (sec. VIII-XIII)* [Milan, 1944], ch. 5; Giorgio Zordan, "I vari aspetti della communione familiare di beni nella Venezia dei secoli XI-XII," *Studi veneziani* 8 (1966): 127-94; Ercole, "Vincende storiche," 410-18.

63. Brandileone, *Scritti di storia,* 302. Justinian first allowed to the poor, widowed partner of a rich spouse one-quarter of the latter's estate (up to 100 pounds of gold), a right he later restricted to undowered widows who had received no *donatio propter nuptias* from their husbands (Turlan, "Recherches sur la quarte").

64. Justinian eventually decreed (V, 3, 20) that the husband's donation could not exceed the dowry. The growing concern for the donation in imperial legislation probably shows considerable Greek influence (Anné, *Les rites des fiançailles*), but its rise also seems to have satisfied social needs, not only in Europe but throughout the Empire. In Byzantine documents a relation between the husband's donation and earlier bridewealth is suggested by the gift's name: *phthorian hednon* (Raphael Taubenschlag, *The Law of Greco-Roman Egypt in the Light of the Papyri, 332 B.C.-640 A.D.* [New York, 1944], 1:96). T. Mommsen and Paul M. Meyer, eds., *Leges novellae ad Theodosianum pertinentes,* 2d ed. (Berlin, 1954), 165; Raymond Monier, *Manuel êlêmentaire de droit romain,* 2 vols., 6th ed. (Darmstadt, 1970, reprint), 1:292-302.

65. Brunner, *Abhandlungen zur Rechtsgeschichte,* 2:80; Percy Corbett, *The Roman Law of Marriage* (Oxford, 1930), 205-7.

66. Since Teutberga's reputed incest with her brother was said to have been sodomitic, a virgin conception achieved by occult practices completed the charges, charges whose truth Teutberga later acknowledged. But her admission, which was believed forced, did not lose her the support of Hincmar or of Pope Nicholas. A full, and still standard, account of the political implications of the case is that of Parisot (Robert Parisot, *Le royaume de Lorraine sous les Carolingiens, 843-923* [Paris, 1898]).

67. Hincmar of Reims, *De divortio Lotharii regis et Teutberga reginae,* in J.P. Migne, ed., Patralogia Latina, 126 (Paris, 1879) 618-619, 648-650; *Epistolae,* in *ibid.,* XXII, 134-143. The presence or absence of *morgengabe* runs as a refrain through this complex case. Adventus of Metz argued, for example, that Lothair had actually been married to Waldralda because his father had given him 100 *mansi* to be used as his husband's gift (*Epis-*

tolae Nicolae I papae, 215). Hincmar argued that in the case of an unconsummated union, the girls' family should be recompensed by being allowed to keep the husband's gift.

68. Merêa, *Estudos de direito hispanico medieval,* 1: docs. 3-4, 8, 12, 17, etc. Ubaldo Pasqui, ed., *Documenti per la storia della città di Arezzo,* 2 vols. (Florence, 1899), 1:198-99. Zordan, "I vari aspetti della commune familiare." Justinian's rules seem to have been unknown in Venice, which clung to the institutions of post-classical Theodosian law. The *donum dei lunae* may have Byzantine origins, being related to the *theoretron,* a gift also awarded in Byzantine Egypt (Taubenschlag, *The Law of Greco-Roman Egypt),* and which was associated among the Greeks with the *pretium pudicitiae.* It was often set at one-twelfth of the woman's dowry, an association that was lost in Venice.

69. Some more recent customs, such as in Augsburg and Basel, would not give *morgengabe* to widows; in some places when it was allowed to widows it was called *abendgabe* (Jean Brissaud, *A History of French Private Law,* trans. Rapelye Howell [Boston, 1912], 754).

70. By the time of the law codes, the right of *Raubehe,* if it had ever existed among the Germans, had been considerably modified; see for contrary arguments Köstler (*Raub-, Kauf-, und Fredelehe*) and Kalifa (*Singularités martrimoniales*). Visigothic law seems to have gone furthest in explicitly denying such a right: the abductor who had forced intercourse on his victim could be enslaved to the woman or her parents (III:3.1,2), and if by mutual agreement marriage was arranged between them, no composition was paid (III:3.7; King, *Law and Society* , 232-3). Among the Burgundians the law of Gundobad provided that an abductor was to pay nine times the "pretium" set for his victim (or six times if she was returned uncorrupted.); in the case of a willing victim, when marriage was generally envisioned, the abductor paid three times the marriage price (or 150 solidi of gold in the case of the highest classes (12, 1-4). A later redaction of the law reduced the compensation paid by the abductors of Burgundian women to the brideprice (61; Hubé, "Histoire de la formation de la loi bourguignonne," 238). Among the Lombards, Rothair (191) set 900 solidi, three times the *wergeld* of the highest class and its brideprice [*meta*] (Liutprand, 62.VIII; 89.VI) as the composition for the abduction of a betrothed woman, after which the abductor might acquire her *mundium.* Later legislation extended this composition to all abductions of unconsecrated women (Liutprand, 31, II). Rothair had intended that half the composition go to the girl's guardian (*mundwald),* half to the king; but Liutprand decreed (31.II) that in the case of a woman whose *mundwald* was other than her father or brothers, 300 solidi were to be paid to the victim herself.

71. Zeumer, *Formulae merowingici,* 85-6; Lemaire, "La donatio de l'epouse."

72. G. Le Bras, "Mariage," in *Dictionnaire de théologie catholique* 9 (1927): 2043-2123; P. Daudet, *Études sur l'histoire de la jurisdiction matrimoniale* (Paris, 1941).

73. Teresa Maria Vinyoles, *Les Barcelonines a la darrieres de l'etat mitjana (1370-1410)* [Barcelona, 1976], 88. Perhaps even more strikingly, this condition applied not to the old *sponsalitum* or tenth but to the countergift to the dowry, the *escreix.*

74. Gero Dolezalek, ed., *Das Imbreviaturbuch des Erzbischöflichen Gerichtsnotars Hubaldus aus Pisa (Mai bis August 1230)* [Cologne and Vienna, 1969], 132-33.

75. Ercole, "Vincende storiche," 19-49; C. Devic and J. Vaissette, *Histoire générale de Languedoc* (Toulouse, 1872-1894), 5: cols. 568-69; P. de Bonnassie, *La Catalogne du milieu du Xe à la fin du XIe siècle* (Toulouse, 1975), 259-60; Manlio Bellomo, *Ricerche sui rapporti patrimoniali tra coniugi* (Varese, 1961), ch. 3; Jesus Lalinde Abadia, "Los pactos matrimoniales catalones," *Annuario de historia del derecho español* 33 (1963): 180-190; Burgues, *Les garanties de restitution,* ch. 2; P. Ourliac and J. de Malafosse, *Histoire du droit privé*-3: *Le droit familiale* (Paris, 1968), 279-86.

76. Georges Duby, *La société aux XIe et XIIe siècles dans la région mâconnaise* (Paris, 1971), 217; B. Guerard, ed., *Cartulaire de l'abbaye de Saint-Victor de Marseille* (Paris), 1: docs. 65, 189, 704; Hilaire, *Le régime des biens* 1:1.

77. Lalinde Abadia, "Los pactos matrimoniales catalones," 162. Mir de Mollet set a further condition of the *sponsalitium:* if his wife predeceased him he had the right to repurchase the fief for 500 morabiti. In the same charter, he acknowledged that his father-in-law

had contributed 200 morabiti to the marriage; but the nature of this gift is not known (ibid., 25-51).

78. *Monumenta Historiae Patriae* 16: Leges Municipales (Turin), 2:1144-50; Bellomo, *Richerche sui rapporti patrimoniali,* 6-7.

79. A. Lattes, *Il diritto consuetudinario delle città lombarde* (Milan, 1899), 420, 446-47.

80. Cesare Imperiale di Sant'Angelo, ed., *Codice diplomatico* (Rome, 1936-1943), 1:153; Diane O. Hughes, "Urban Growth and Family Structure in Medieval Genoa," *Past & Present* 66 (1975): 14-15.

81. L. Belgrano and C. Imperiale di Sant'Angelo, eds., *Annali genovesi di Caffaro e de' suoi continuatori* (Rome, 1890-1929), 2:31.

82. M. Chiaudano and M. Moresco, eds., *Il cartolare di Giovanni Scriba* (Genoa, 1935), no. 376.

83. Brandileone, *Scritti di storia,* 308-11; Bellomo, *Ricerche sui rapporti patrimoniali,* chap. 1. One rather surprising exception is Savona where *quarta* was allowed to childless widows; but it could not exceed 50 pounds, and was clearly intended to provide for poorer women (Laura Balletto, ed., *Statuta antiquissima Saone (1345)* [Bordighera, 1971], 2:182-83).

84. Bellomo, *Ricerche sui rapporti patrimoniali,* chap. 8.

85. Geneviève Laribière, "Le mariage à Toulouse aux XIVe et XVe siècles," *Annales du Midi* 79 (1967): 335-61; Hilaire, *Le régime des biens* 1:3.

86. Where there is some evidence of its existence at the turn of the century (Barcelona, A.C. Div. B 913 [in the possession of a wife in 1299], 1783 [its award with *sponsalitium* in 1209]).

87. Lalinde Abadia, *Los pactos matrimoniales,* 249-50, 252-53.

88. Barcelona, A.C. Div. B 1783.

89. A. Aunos Perez, *El derecho catalan en el siglo XIII* (Barcelona, 1926), 1; Vinyoles, *Barcelonines,* 88-89. In Barcelona, however, the *escreix* seems to have been tied only to the assessed dowry *(dos estimata)*. Unassessed lands and real estate were not met with counterdower.

90. Barcelona, A.C. Div. A 2012; Lalinde Abadia, *Los pactos matrimoniales,* 255-56.

91. Archívo Histórico de Protocólos de Barcelona, Pere Portel, *Manuel* (1299), ff. 67-68.

92. Goody and Tambiah, *Bridewealth and Dowry,* 64.

93. Strictly speaking, the Roman dowry did not represent a daughter's share of her paternal inheritance; but there are signs that by late imperial times fathers were coming to regard the award of a dowry as a daughter's chief claim on their estates (H.J. Wolff, "Zur Stellung der Frau im klassischen romischen Dotalrecht," *Zeitschrift der Savigny-Stiftung fur Rechtsgeschichte* Rom. Abt. 53 [1933]: 297-371), as it was in Greece (Wolff, "Marriage Law and Family Organization in Ancient Athens," *Traditio* 2 [1944]: 43-95).

94. F. Bonsini, ed., *Constituta legis et usus pisanae civitatis* (Florence, 1870), 2:745; Bellomo, *Ricerche sui rapporti patrimoniali,* chap. 6; A. Pertile, *Storia del diritto italiano,* 6 vols., 2d ed. (Bologna, 1966), 4:58.

95. *Leges Langobardorum,* Edictum Rotharii, 181; Liutprand 2.1; Lattes, *Il diritto consuetudinario,* 259. Some historians have traced the roots of this exclusion to Greco-Roman law, which influenced Italian maritime cities (P.S. Leicht, *Scritti vari di storia del diritto italiano,* 2 vols. [Milan, 1948], 2:194 ff.).

96. N. Didier, "Les dispositions du statut de Guillaume II de Forcalquier sur les filles dotées (1162)," *Le Moyen-Age* 56 (1950): 255, nn. 34-36; 266-67; P.C. Timbal, "La devolution sucessorale 'ab intestat' dans la coutume de Toulouse," *Revue historique de droit français et étranger* 4th ser., 33 (1955): 77; R. Aubenas, *Cours d'histoire du droit privé,* 6 vols. (Aix-en-Provence, 1954-1958), 3.

97. Bonnassie, *La Catalogne,* 260 n. 11.

98. J. Ruis Serra, ed., *Cartulario de Sant Cujat del Vallés,* 3 vols. (Barcelona, 1946), 3: 979. So too, Ramón de Odena, in his will of 1196, left landed wealth to his two sons,

whom he charged to pay 500 morabiti to marry one of their sisters. The other he committed to the nunnery (Cartulario de S. Cujat, 3:215). When Catalonian fathers did still leave their married daughters real legacies, it was often in the face of irregular family situations. Guillermo de. S. Oliva left his married daughter a fortress in 1226, for example; but she received it because his only sons were "spuru et dampnato coitu procreati," for although he had married their mother "in faciam ecclesie" and had received from her 12,000 solidi (presumably as dowry), the union was bigamous since she already had a living husband (ibid, 3:1301).

99. Guillermo de Broca, *Historia del derecho de Cataluña* (Barcelona; 1918) 1:261.

100. Aubenas, *Cours d'historie*, 3. D. Hughes, "Struttura familiare e sistemi di successione ereditaria nei testamenti dell'Europa medievale," *Quaderni storici* 33 (1976): 938.

101. Ibid., 943-5.

102. Didier, "Les dispositions," 252.

103. In Genoa, as elsewhere in Italy, daughters were admitted to "legitima" (usually a share of the one-quarter of the estate that was reserved for the natural heirs) in their parents' estate, although the dowry was calculated in this amount (C. Desimoni and A. Belgrano, eds., *Leges genuenses* [Turin; 1901] 18: cols. 893-5). Such a right was strongly argued for—against the "favor masculorum et agnationis"—in the later Middle Ages in Savoy when statutes began to limit the value of dowries (Maria Benedetto, *Ricerche sui rapporti patrimoniali tra coniugi nello stato sabaudo* [Turin, 1957], 91). But in many places throughout the south the right to a "legitima" was explicitly denied (Didier, "Les dispositions," 275; Timbal, "La dévolution successorale," 77).

104. Enrico Fiumi, ed., *Statuti di Volterra* (Florence; 1952), 10; L. Frati, ed., *Statuti di Bologna dall'anno 1245 all'anno 1267* (Bologna,1869), 1:414-5.

105. *Liber instrumentorum, Cartulaire des Guillems de Montpellier* (Montpellier, 1884-1886), 184-9. The heir in reserve (often named William in anticipation of the death of the first son) was generally granted little land but was awarded an annual income; those destined for the Church received, like their sisters, a cash settlement (*Liber instrumentorum*, 177-89, 195-206).

106. Archivio di Stato, Genoa, Sez. notarile, Cartulary of Simone Vataccio, 3:ii, ff. 66, 69v, 74v, 76r; R.S. Lopez, "Familiari, procuratori e dipendenti di Benedetto Zaccaria," *Miscellanea di storia ligure in onore di Giorgia Falco* (Milan, 1962), 225-26.

107. M. Chiaudano and R. della Rocca, eds., *Oberto Scriba de Mercato (1190)* [Genoa, 1938], nos. 502-3.

108. E. Ricotti, ed., *Liber jurium reipublicae genuensis* 7 (Turin, 1854), cols. 679-82.

109. Decretales, V.19.16; A Potthast, *Regesta pontificum Romanorum* (Berlin, 1874), 1:5038.

110. Didier, "Les dispositions," 258, n. 53.

111. Devic and Vaissette, *Histoire générale de Languedoc* 5:257-58, 886, 889-94; *Liber instrumentorum*, 339-40, 349-52.

112. R. Aubenas, *Le testament en Provence dans l'ancien droit* (Aix-en-Provence, 1927), 8-9.

113. Hilaire, *Le régime des biens* 1:1; Barcelona A.C. Div. A 2012, 2177; Portell, *Manuel*, ff. 67r-68r, 101.

114. See Eleanor Riemer's article in this volume, "Women, Dowries and Capital Investment in Thirteenth Century Siena," p. 65; Laribière, "Le mariage à Toulouse." Sometimes the cash settlement covered a trousseau of clothes and of household items, which were not necessarily described; property, however, seems almost always to have been separately described even when it was assigned a cash value.

115. Hilaire, *Le régime des biens*, 59-60.

116. G. de Bonnecorse de Lubières, *La condition des gens mariés en Provence aux XIVe, XVe, XVIe siècles* (Paris, 1929), 144-66.

117. P. Santini, *Documenti dell'antica costituzione del comune di Firenze* (Florence, 1895), 530.

118. Bonnecorse de Lubieres, *La condition des gens mariés*, 149-62.

119. Archivo Historico de Protocolos de Barcelona, Pere Portell, *Manuel* (1299), ff. 67r-68v; Berenguer Ermengol, *Manuel* (1381-1382), ff. 107r. It would be interesting to know how common this practice was. In Anjou a charter from 1155 describes property that descended as dowry within the female line through successive generations. (Penny Gold, "Image and Reality: Women in Twelfth-Century France." [PhD. dissertation, Stanford University, 1977], 257-58, n. 93).

120. Initially, of course, in a Roman marriage *cum manu,* the wife's dowry had fallen totally within her husband's control. By Cicero's day, however, women *in manu* had the same rights of recovery of dowry as wives of free marriages, and these rights became more extensive as a result of later imperial legislation (Corbett, *The Roman Law of Marriage;* Wolff, "Zur Stellung der Frau").

121. Hilaire, *Le regime des biens,* I.1; Burgues, *Les garanties de restitution,* ch. 1.

122. Monier, *Manuel élêmentaire de droit romain,* I:291.

123. Burgues, *Les garanties de restitution,* chap. 1.

124. Aubenas, *Cours d'histoire* II:35-6.

125. Ermengol, *Manuel,* ff.107v-108r.

126. A. M. Visdominus, ed. *Statuta et decreta comunis Genuae* (Bologna; 1498), 25.

127. Bellomo, *Ricerche sui rapporti patrimoniali,* chap. 7.

128. Barcelona, Archiv Capilular, Div. A 2280b.

129. *Statuta et decreta comunis Genuae,* 36v; Vaccari, *Scritti di storia,* 140. A similar system in Siena awarded widowers a stated "lucro" of their wives' dowries; this was also the amount widows might claim as their "lucro donationis." But the amounts involved were significantly smaller: in the first half of the thirteenth century the average dowry was 100 lire but over half the *lucri* awarded were less than one-fifth of that amount, and fully 36 percent were 100 solidi. This was, moreover, a percentage that declined in the last half of the century when the average dowry rose to 205 lire but the *lucro* remained substantially the same (Eleanor Riemer, "Women in the Medieval City: Sources and Uses of Wealth by Sienese Women in the Thirteenth Century" [PhD. dissertation, New York University, 1975], 93-95, figs. 5,6).

130. Louis de Charrin, *Les testaments dans la région de Montpellier au Moyen Age* (Ambilly, 1961), 100-101; Hilaire, *Le régime des biens* 2:1; Aubenas, *Cours d'histoire* 1:37; Burgues, *Les garanties de restitution,* chap. 1.

131. A. Aúnos Perez, *El derecho catalan,* 1.

132. E. de Hinojosa, "La reception du droit romain en Catalogne," in *Mélanges Fitting* (1969, reprint), 2:391-408. It seems to have penetrated Catalonia after neighboring Septimania. The appearance of the will has often been taken as a sign of Roman legal influence, and it was popular in Catalonia decades before it attained stature elsewhere along the northern Mediterranean littoral (Carlin, *Le testament en Provence,* 66-68). But the will in Catalonia generally antedates the acceptance of other Roman legal forms and should probably be seen as a Visigothic survival (J. Bastier, "Le testament en Catalogne du IXe au XIIe siècle: une survivance wisigothique," *Revue de droit français et étranger* 4th ser., 51 (1973): 373-417.

133. Lalinde Abadia, *Los pactos matrimoniales,* 102.

134. A Finocchiaro Sartorio. *La communione dei beni tre coniugi nella stori del diritto italiano* (Palermo, 1902); Toubert, *Les structures du Latium médiéval,* 762-63.

135. D.O. Hughes, "Urban Growth and Family Structure," 24; "Domestic Ideals and Social Behavior: Evidence from Medieval Genoa," in Charles Rosenberg, ed., *The Family in History* (Philadelphia, 1975), 129-30.

136. D. Bizzari, *Studi di storia del diritto italiano* (Turin, 1937), 248.

137. I describe this in some detail in my forthcoming book, *Marriage and Social Change in Three Mediterranean Countries: Genoa, Marseille, Barcelona, 1150-1450,* which is based largely on analysis of notarial records.

138. *Decretum.* C.31 q.2 c.1; J. Noonan, "Power to Choose," *Viator* 4 (1973): 419-35; Le Bras, "Mariage," *Dictionnaire de théologie catholique.*

139. *Statuta et decreta comunis Genuae:* 25v; Aubenas, *Cours d'histoire;* Vinyoles, *Les Barcelonines,* 102-3.

140. G. Stella, *Annales genuenses,* G.P. Balbi, ed. (Bologna, 1975), 118.

141. Vinyoles, *Les Barcelonines,* 168-169.

142. J.M. Vidal, ed., *Lettres communes,* 3 vols., (Rome, 1902-1911), no. 7208. Such dispensation for marriage to a consanguine or affine who took in marriage an undowered woman or who gave her dowry from his goods was canonical (Al. de Smet, *Tractatus theologico-canonicis de sponsalibus et matrimonio,* 4th ed. (Bruges, 1927), 685.

143. *Leges Langobardorum,* Liutprand, 117.I; 129.XIII; Aistulf, 10.I.

144. Hughes, "Urban Growth and Family Structure," 18, 27.

145. M. Hasluck, "Bride-Price in Albania: A Homeric Parallel," *Man* 33 (1933): 191-95.

146. Alain de Lille, *The Complaint of Nature,* trans. Douglas M. Moffat (New York, 1908), 55; D. Herlihy, "The Generation in Medieval History," *Viator* 5 (1974): 362; "Life Expectancies for Women in the Middle Ages," in *The Role of Women in the Middle Ages,* Rosemarie Morewedge, ed. (Albany, 1975).

147. Walter K. Lacey, *The Family in Classical Greece* (Ithaca, N.Y., 1968), 205; Hasluck, *Bride-Price in Albania.* Aristotle had proposed a reverse argument for Sparta; namely, that the award of vast dowries and a related tendency to allow heiresses had put two-fifths of the country in the hands of a small number of women and had so impoverished Sparta's men that "while the territory would have supported 1500 horse and 30,000 foot, the number had dwindled to less than 1000" (*Politics* 2, ix 1270 a 16). Hasluck's suggestion (almost immediately rejected by Myres [J.A.L. Myres, "Homeric and Albanian Bride-Price," *Man* 33 (1933):195-96]), that the shift into dowry marriage in ancient Greece was linked to the large-scale colonization that swept post-Homeric Greece, taking prospective bridegrooms far away from home, was an extension of her explanation of a modern Albanian situation.

148. It is based largely on demographic evidence contained in Carolingian polyptychs, whose low female population has always been regarded with suspicion—although one must now take into account the hypothesis of Coleman (Emily R. Coleman, "L'infanticide dans le Haut Moyen Age," *Annales* E.S.C. 29 (1974), 315-35). It should be noted, however, that at Saint-Germain des Prés, in spite of an extraordinarily high sex ratio, many adult women remained unmarried, perhaps kept single, as Coleman suggested (p. 333), because the land would not support further households. It would be wrong, furthermore, to take the high sex ratio at Saint-Germain as typical of the Carolingian world. The polyptych of Saint Victor of Marseille, for example, reveals the existence there of 106 girls and 99 boys (B. Guerard, ed. *Cartulaire de l'abbaye de Saint-Victor de Marseille* [Paris], 633-56; Coleman, "Medieval Marriage Characteristics," 330). Finally, the value of the polyptychs is limited by the fact that they survey a tenant population, the exposure of whose adult men to violent death was less of a threat than among the free Germanic population about whose marriage settlements the codes legislate. Indeed, Kalifa supposes this to have been so high that excess women would submit to marriage by seizure ("Singularités matrimoniales," 225); but this seems an equally shaky hypothesis.

149. *Leges Langobardorum,* Aistulf 10.I; Edictum Rotharii, 221; Ratchis 6.II. Some eighth-century charters suggest, furthermore, that this may have been a common practice (Schiaparelli, *Codice diplomatico Langobardo* 1:29, 53, 55). One encounters a similar tendency on the estates of Saint Germain at the beginning of the ninth century. There, however, the penalties were less severe, for the children took their mother's status (E. Coleman, "Medieval Marriage Characteristics: A Neglected Factor in the History of Medieval Serfdom," *Journal of Interdisciplinary History* 2 [1971]: 205-19).

150. King Liutprand did forbid in 731 (*Leges Langobardorum,* Liutprand, 129.XIII) a "perversion" that had appeared among the Lombards in his day: the union of adult women with boys who had not attained puberty (that is, they were under 14 years of age). He speaks of the boys as fatherless, and it seems clear that their value lay in the estate they commanded. It is impossible to know how prevalent such a practice may have been; but, of course, it is in striking contrast to the urban legislation from the later Middle Ages, which concerned itself with the marriage of prenubile girls.

151. P. Bonnassie, "Une famille de la campagne barcelonaise et ses activités economiques aux alentours de l'An Mil," *Annales du Midi* 7 (1964):259.

152. *Liber instrumentorum,* 177-89, 193-206, 240-1. For every three sons that probably had a sufficiency for marriage, four daughters were awarded dowries; no single father seems to have been willing, however, to dower more than three daughters: the others were made nuns.

153. A fairly significant difference in marriage age has been found between men and women in fifteenth-century Florence (Herlihy, "Mapping Households in Medieval Italy," *Catholic Historical Review* 58 [1972]: 14), for example; and a similar discrepancy has been postulated in southern France, where it may have led to the expansion and semi-institutionalization of prostitution (J. Roussiaud, "Prostitution, jeunesse et société dans les villes du Sud-Est au XVe siècle," *Annales* E.S.C. 31 [1976]:3. In other places, such as medieval Genoa, however, all men seem to have married at a reasonably early age, especially within the urban patriciate.

154. *Leges Langobardorum,* Liutprand, 1.I.

155. Ibid, 14.I. This reversed Liutprand 103.VIII; the charters record some illegal grants of usufruct to wives before Aistulf altered the law, and after that time men began regularly to award usufruct in their estate to their wives, usually on condition that they remain widows (Schiaparelli, *Codice diplomatico Langobardo* 1:82; 2:281, 287, 293). Aistulf limited this right if the match had produced children: in that case a man might only award his widow usufruct of one-half of his estate (or less in the case of additional children from previous marriages).

156. And within the conjugal family what should be stressed is the rough equality and independence of husband and wife—not only in the familial economy but also in the cognatic kinship and inheritance systems that underlay it.

157. Duby, *La société dans la region mâconnaise,* 263-81; D. Herlihy, "Family solidarity in Medieval Italian History," in David Herlihy, Robert S. Lopez and Vsevolod Slessarev, eds., *Economy, Society and Government* [Kent, Ohio, 1969]; Hughes, "Urban Growth and Family Structure".

158. Perhaps increased obedience to principles of exogamy did distinguish later from early medieval marriage. The frequency of cousin, and especially uncle-niece marriage among landowning families in Spain in the early Middle Ages (E. Saez, "Los ascendientes de San Rosendo," *Hispania* 8 [1948]:3-76; M. del Carmen Carle, "Gran propriedad y grandes proprietarios," *Cuadernos de historia* de Espana 77-8 [1973]: 53-56) is probably not a uniquely Iberian phenomenon.

159. Devic and Vaissette, *Histoire génêrale de Languedoc* 5; 1171-74.

160. Belgrano, *Della vita privata dei genovesi,* 393-405.

161. *Paradiso* 15:103-5.

162. J.P. Cooper, "Patterns of Inheritance and Settlement by Great Landowners from the Fifteenth to the Eighteenth Centuries," in Jack Goody, Joan Thirsk and E.P. Thompson, eds., *Family and Inheritance: Rural Society in Western Europe, 1200-1800* (Cambridge; 1976), 192-312; M. Petitjean, *Essai sur l'histoire des substitutions du IXe au XVe siècle dans la pratique et la doctrine, spécialement en France méridionale* (Dijon, 1975).

163. D. Puncuh, "La vita savonese agli inizi del Duecento," in *Miscellanea di Storia ligure in onore di Giorgio Falco* (Milan, 1962), 132.

164. J.K. Hyde, *Padua in the Age of Dante* (Manchester, 1966), 140-41.

165. G.A. Brucker, *Renaissance Florence* (New York, 1969), 92-93.

166. S. Chojnacki, "Dowries and Kinsmen in Early Renaissance Venice," *Journal of Interdisciplinary History* 5 (1975): 571-600. In Genoa, however, aristocratic women seem not to have contributed with such fervor to the dowries of their kinswomen.

167. Cooper, "Patterns of Inheritance and Settlement."

168. Such a marital regime created a community between the spouses and can be found throughout the dotal South in the later Middle Ages. It was part of larger experiments with various kinds of *fraternitas,* which joined both kinsmen and strangers into a household community (R. Aubenas, "Le contrat d'affrairamentum dans le droit provençal du Moyen Age,"

Revue historique de droit français et étranger 4th ser., 12 (1933): 478-524; "Tendances archaisantes et famille artificielle en pays de droit écrit au Moyen Age," *Annales du Midi* 53(1941): 113-41; "Reflections sur les 'fraternités artificielles au Moyen Age," in *Études d'histoire à la memoire de Noël Didier* [Paris, 1961], 1-10; J. Gaudemet, "Les communautés familiales," [Paris, 1965]), 84-131).

169. The *albergo* was a formal union of (related and unrelated) aristocratic families who shared the same urban space. Although their formation can be traced in Genoa as early as the thirteenth century, they developed most rapidly in the late fourteenth and early fifteenth centuries (E. Grendi, "Profilo storico degli alberghi genovesi," *Mélanges de l'École française de Rome,* 87 [1975], Hughes, "Kinsmen and Neighbors in Medieval Genoa," in H.A. Miskimin, D. Herlihy, and A.L. Udovitch, eds., *The Medieval City* [New Haven, 1977], 95-111).

170. G. Saige, ed., *Documents historiques relatifs à la principauté de Monaco depuis le quinzième siècle* (Monaco, 1888) 1:236-43, 268-73, 609-22.

171. N. Battilana, *Genealogia delle famiglie nobili di Genova,* (Genoa, 1825-1833); Archivio Stato, Genoa, Sezione Notarile, Oberto Foglietta, Jr., Filza 1 (1436-1449), ff. 163, 204, 357. Violantina's domestic strength was undeniable; when her husband made a will in 1439 naming his brother heir in the absence of children, it was promptly revoked in her favor; and her father, rather than his brother, was named as tutor to any children the couple might have.

172. C. Grimaldi, *Mémoires de Charles Grimaldi, marquis de Regusse, 1612-65* (Aix-en-Provence, 1870), 4.

173. Lawrence Stone, *The Crisis of the Aristocracy* (Oxford, 1965), 632-45.

174. In some places, of course, the delayed marriage of men and early marriage of women may have produced a similar effect.

175. N. Yalman, *Under the Bo Tree: Studies in Caste, Kinship and Marriage in the Interior of Ceylon* (Berkeley, 1967), 172-7. J.L. McCreery, "Women's Property Rights and Dowry in China and South Asia," *Ethnology* 15 (1976): 163-74.

176. A. de Leone and A. Piccirillo, eds., *Consuetudines civitatis Amalfie* (Naples, 1970), 48. But all widows with children were allowed rights in a part of their husbands' estates equal to the part of each of their children.

177. Lalinde Abadia, "Los pactos matrimoniales," 260-6.

178. The first examples of running the gauntlet, whose origins some would trace to ancient Germanic practice, come from southern France in the early decades of the thirteenth century; but by the latter half of the century, a fine was regularly proposed as an alternative (Aubenas, *Cours d'histoire* 6:55-7). In the fourteenth century some examples have been found of an actual running, but by the fifteenth century payment came to be preferred (ibid., 59-60).

Women, Dowries, and Capital Investment in Thirteenth-Century Siena

Eleanor S. Riemer

It is now almost a commonplace among historians of women that conventional notions of "progress" will not withstand the scrutiny of feminist scholarship. Not only has progress often meant different things for women and men, but in many periods, the conditions which brought economic, political, or intellectual advancement for men—or at least certain classes of men—had the reverse effect on women. Perhaps no one has made this point more eloquently than Joan Kelly, whose groundbreaking study asked: "Did women have a Renaissance?," and concluded: "no"—"at least not during the Renaissance."[1]

Although the denial of social and economic rights and prerogatives to women is readily apparent by the early modern period, we do not yet know the exact moment when women first began to lose ground (if indeed there was "one moment"), nor precisely how it happened. One reason is that the transformations in the social and economic structure which so significantly altered women's and men's lives occurred unevenly across Europe and at different times—from what is conventionally called the late middle ages through the early modern centuries. So, as Joan Kelly believed, if we are to adequately understand the phenomenon of retrenchment for women, we must make detailed studies of specific groups of European women to determine when and under what circumstances their status and roles were altered.

This is a case study of middle- and upper-class women in Siena, Italy during the thirteenth and early fourteenth centuries. This was the age in Siena of the great burgeoning of commercial capitalism which affected every level—and gender—of society. Women, in this period, experienced first an expansion of their legal prerogatives and economic opportunities, and then their erosion.

I have drawn on the extensive notarial evidence available for this period (especially pre-nuptual property settlements, conveyences of property, and wills) and the law codes of 1256 and 1309-10 to show: first, that by the beginning of the thirteenth century, Sienese women enjoyed considerable rights over property and their own persons, rights which were protected by law; second, that middle- and upper-class women used their prerogatives to take advantage of the opportunities offered by the developing commercial capitalism of the thirteenth century and, moreover, did so in ways that threatened male economic and lineal interests; and, third, male reaction to women's independent economic activity resulted in the constriction of women's rights, specifically, their ability to control capital.

The dowry played a key role in this process. It provided a bridge between women's "traditional" status in the family and their roles in the new economy. It was through the dowry, which in this period was transformed from a payment in property to a payment in cash, that women received substantial amounts of capital: it was women's free use of this capital that men sought to curb.

During the thirteenth century, the city-republic of Siena underwent a profound, some scholars say "precocious," commercial growth and development.[2] The lines of the economy were reshaped as commerce (both local and international) and banking gained in scope and importance. The increased variety and volume of commercial opportunities and the accompanying accumulation of wealth greatly altered the life of the Sienese, most notably of the men of the upper and middle classes. These "citizens and merchants," who held political and economic power, devoted ever greater amounts of capital to trade, loans, and exchange as the century progressed. As commercial activity and the amount of cash in circulation increased, so did the opportunities even for small investors, to participate in new types of commercial and speculative ventures.[3] These activities were not confined to men: by the beginning of the thirteenth century, upper- and middle-class Sienese women had begun to take advantage of the expanding commercial opportunities.

By the thirteenth century Sienese women had considerable freedom of action and legal responsibilities. Some scholars have attributed this to the Commune's adoption of Roman law in place of Lombard law in 1176. As a result, from the late twelfth century, Sienese women were no longer subject to the guardianship (*mundium*) of fathers and husbands as they had been under the germanic codes, and in most cases could conduct their own legal and economic affairs.[4] Married and unmarried women could inherit and dispose of property, enter into contracts, assume financial obligations, buy and sell real estate and other goods, lend money, sue and be sued, and give surety. They could plead their own cases in court or name someone to do it for them. Women could draw up wills, make donations to charitable and religious institutions, and give gifts to individuals. A woman could assume the guardianship of her children when her husband died.[5]

As a result of these rights and liberties and the opportunities offered by the new commercial economy, Sienese women—single, married, and widowed—engaged in a wide variety of economic activities in the thirteenth century. These included those which might be characterized as "traditional" in medieval society, i.e., widows selling land in conjunction with male relatives, as well as commercial ventures which were part of the new economic order, such as lending money as an investment. Notarial contracts from this period frequently showed women, married and unmarried, purchasing and selling real estate.[6] Women also rented out shops in the city and land in the countryside,[7] and sold the grain and other products of their land.[8]

One of the most interesting commercial activities women engaged in was moneychanging. Even in the early thirteenth century, women were involved, albeit in a minor way, in the exchange of currencies.[9] Women also lent money, which, in the Sienese economy, was often a form of business investment.[10] In the contracts which recorded these transactions, the debtor declared himself and his firm (*società*) in debt to the woman for the amount of the loan which he promised to repay on a specified date.[11]

Women also performed the important function of granting surety, both for men and for other women.[12] Documents from as early as the 1220s show women, both married and single, providing surety for men, including some who did not appear to be relatives, in matters such as loans and the sale of cloth.[13]

A detailed picture of the activities of women during the first part of the century can be found in two notaries' notebooks, one for the years 1221-23, the other for 1227-28.[14] While the number of women's commercial documents in these notebooks is small (40 out of 390 in 1221-23 and 27 out of 223 in 1227-29) they clearly show that, even in those early years, women engaged in a variety of speculative and commercial activities independently of men.

In these notebooks the most numerous and important kinds of ventures for women were loans, currency exchanges, and sales of goods for local consumption.[15] Moneylending played a large role in women's activities; the sums women lent varied from as little as 20 *soldi* to as much as £ 200.[16] Most interestingly, women usually lent money without the formal consent or partnership of men; indeed, they were more likely to undertake commercial ventures alone or in association with other women than transactions involving real estate. When land was involved, especially its sale or permanent alienation by a female owner, the woman involved was most likely to appear in the contract as a coseller with men—usually one or more male relatives.[17] Clearly, women did not deal as freely and independently with this traditional source of wealth, which was still the foundation of many families' patrimonies, as they did with the new forms derived from commerce and moneylending.

Of course, women's rights and prerogatives were hardly equal to men's. The Sienese legal codes were based on juridical principles which relegated women to a secondary position in society and thirteenth-century legislation reinforced women's disabilities. Nowhere is this clearer than in the laws governing inheritance: males and the male line were consistently favored in the devolution of real and personal property.[18] For example, while the legal codes recognized the validity of wills made by women and men[19] and, therefore, women's ability to inherit property based on testamentary bequests, the codes stipulated that male relatives were to take precedence over females when the deceased died intestate.[20] Perhaps the most striking example in the statutes of the preference for males is the exclusion of a dowered daughter from any share in both her father's and mother's estates when the parents died intestate and were survived by sons.[21] A daughter's dowry was her share of the patrimony; she was entitled to nothing more. All the family's remaining property was to pass to sons.

The exclusion of dowered daughters from paternal inheritance (the *exclusio propter dotem*) was common throughout Italy in the thirteenth century,[22] but the Sienese legislation went further than that of other cities by barring daughters from maternal inheritance as well and in stipulating that the exclusion held even when the dowry had been provided by family members other than the parents. To further ensure that property passed in the male lineage, the exclusion was extended to a dowered daughter's heirs if legitimate off-spring of sons survived.

While women's property rights were limited, they were also specifically defined and protected by law. Most important was the protection of a woman's rights over her dowry. From the second half of the twelfth century the Sienese employed the late Roman (actually Code Justinian) system of marriage exchange, with the dowry (*dos*) given by the bride's father to the groom as its keystone.[23] While the husband had the use of the dowry for the duration of the marriage, law and custom considered it the wife's property, to be returned to her when the marriage ended.[24] To ensure that a woman would not be coerced into giving her dowry outright to her husband, a statute forbade her from doing so without the consent of "three close relatives" who, presumably, would defend her interests against a greedy husband.[25]

Other statutory safeguards sought to ensure the dowry's return to a widow after her husband's death. A wife held a mortgage (*ypoteca*) on her husband's property for the amount of her dowry. She was his first creditor and had to be paid before other debts were settled from his estate.[26] In addition, the law codes made specific provisions for the restitution of the dowry to a widow by her husband's heirs (usually his sons). They had a specified time in which to settle the estate and pay the widow what she was owed; until then they were required to provide her with food, clothing, and shelter.[27] Although a woman could waive restitution and live with and be supported by her sons, she had the right to go to court and insist that her dowry be restored to her. Once she did this, her children had to pay up within two months.[28] From the middle of the thirteenth century women had recourse to the Curia del Placito, a court whose function was to oversee the property rights of women and minors.[29]

In the thirteenth century, then, Sienese women had the legal ability to acquire, use, and dispose of property and thus take advantage of the century's expanding commercial opportunities. Of course, a woman's ability to participate in the new economic order was contingent upon her having the capital with which to do so—and many women did. Although dowered daughters were barred from intestate succession to their parents' estates, any woman could be the beneficiary of a testamentary bequest and could also receive gifts from living individuals. In fact, fathers, mothers, and husbands, as well as brothers, grandparents, and other relatives and friends made bequests and gave gifts to their female relatives and friends. But fathers and husbands, who controlled most of their families' wealth, did not leave significant amounts of cash or property to their daughters or wives. While many fathers provided for their unmarried daughters' dowries in their wills, few left them or their married sisters any additional legacies, and when they did, the amounts were small.[30] Husbands frequently made bequests to their wives, but they, too, were small, generally consisting of the woman's own clothing and jewelry, a small sum in cash, or occasionally a small annuity. Moreover, conditions were often attached to these meager bequests, such as that the widow remain in her husband's house and not ask that her dowry be restored.[31] Presumably her sons, who could then keep the dowry, would support her. Other husbands were more specific in their attempts to control their wives' economic and sexual lives from the grave, like the man who stipulated that his wife could keep her inheritance only if she lived "without a man, chaste, and unmarried."[32]

The most regular and valuable source of capital for women, then, was their dowries. We must therefore look more closely at the dowry and the nature of Sienese prenuptual property settlements to understand how women acquired the major portion of their wealth and how they may have used it for their own purposes.

It was universally accepted among the Sienese that every woman must have a dowry; not only fathers, but brothers, mothers, sisters, grandfathers, uncles, and sometimes more distant relatives provided brides' dowries or made contributions to them.[33] Guardians of orphaned girls saw that their charges received adequate dowries[34] and some grandfathers made provisions for their as yet unborn granddaughters in their wills.[35] The government itself apparently considered the dowry one of the necessities of life, since it allowed the amount of a dowry assigned to a daughter to be deducted, along with expenses for food, furniture and clothing, from the assessed valuation of a person's taxable property.[36]

The importance of the dowry for marriage exchange and the Sienese economy should not be underestimated. By the thirteenth century, it served a number of purposes, beyond the traditional one of helping the husband "bear the burdens of matrimony."[37] Among the bourgeoisie, marriage alliances often created or cemented business partnerships, so the giving of a dowry often may have served as a business investment for the bride's family. Certainly Sienese bridegrooms looked on the dowry as a major source of their own investment capital.[38] But the dowry had commercial significance for women as well. Although a husband had control over it during the marriage and retained any profits from investing it, the dowry belonged to the wife, who was entitled and expected to come into full possession of it in widowhood. Thus, the dowry was a potential source of investment capital for women, too.

The property settlements between the families of the bride and groom (most often between the groom and the bride's father) were recorded in notarial contracts, hundreds of which survive from the thirteenth and early fourteenth centuries.[39] The contracts usually describe the dowry as a sum of money or property to which a cash value was applied. Occasionally real property without a cash value (*inextimata*) was given, and in some instances a combination of valued (*extimata*) and unvalued property (including real estate) or rights of credit were stipulated.[40] But it appears that by the thirteenth century a dowry was most commonly granted as a specific sum of money, without reference to either real estate or moveable property, a trend noted in other parts of Italy[41] and undoubtedly the result of the burgeoning commercial economy. However, most of the surviving contracts are not those which conferred the dowry, but rather the reciprocal agreement made by the bridegroom (or someone else for him, if he was a minor), and the bride's father, the *donatione propter nuptias.*[42] In Siena, the *donatione* did not represent a payment from the groom to the bride; rather, it was a pledge that a portion of the husband's property, equal in value to the dowry, would be reserved for the wife to ensure that her dowry would be returned to her at his death. It made the wife her husband's first creditor, granting her a mortgage on his property for the amount of her dowry.[43] Thus, in some cases, the dowry itself might have consisted of real and/or personal property, but the *donatione* only referred to its cash value. In fact, at least partial payment occasionally was made in land, houses, vineyards, or other real estate. Yet the evidence suggests that the cash dowry was becoming the norm, and whether or not the entire dowry was given to the groom in cash, it almost always had a cash value.[45]

Cash dowries, which could be used as investment capital, were undoubtedly attractive to bridegrooms and brides' male relatives in thirteenth-century Siena. But the conversion of the dowry into a cash payment may have been spurred on by other considerations. In Siena, as elsewhere in medieval and Renaissance Europe, men sought to limit or prohibit women's ownership of landed property, which, the "commercial revolution" notwithstanding, still had considerable economic importance and symbolic significance for the males of patrilineally defined families. Converting the dowry to cash was one means of preventing landed wealth from passing to females or the families into which they married.[46] Nevertheless, cash dowries and, more importantly, the application of a cash value to dowries, were a boon to women's property rights in late medieval Siena. A woman was assured that the value of her dowry rather than specific property or goods would be restored to her. So even if part of the original dowry was no longer part of her husband's estate when he died, the widow still had a claim on the estate: she could then come into possession of her husband's interests in business ventures, his rights of credit, cash, or real estate in the amount stipulated in the *donatione.*

An examination of 130 dowry and *donatione* contracts (see table 1) reveals how much money women actually received in widowhood. Clearly, the value of dowries rose steadily during the course of the century. In the period 1201-49 the average dowry was £ 100; in the last twenty years of the century, from 1280-99, the average was £ 205, an increase of over 100 percent. A comparison of the range and distribution of dowries between the early and later parts of the century makes the rise even more obvious. In the years 1201-15, the average dowry was £ 35 and all were under £ 60. By the 1240s, the average was £ 149 and only 50 percent were under £ 60. By the last decade of the century the average dowry had risen to £ 215 and only 15 percent were under £ 60. By that time 51 percent were between £ 100 and £ 499 and 10 percent were over £ 500. There were no dowries of £ 1000 or more before 1240, but there were four in the last twenty years of the century.

This sharp increase appears to be part of a pattern of spiralling dowry levels which characterized Italian cities in the late middle ages and Renaissance. Various explanations, none totally satisfactory, have been offered for this phenomenon. One possible cause may have been increased demands by bridegrooms in the face of a soaring cost of living. A traditional purpose of the dowry, after all, was to allow the husband to support his wife. Thus, a general correlation at least might be drawn between the rising cost and standard of living and rising dowry levels.[47] It has also been suggested that demographic changes, specifically a surplus of marriageable females, caused dowries to rise.[48] But the dowry's inflationary spiral might have been directly related to the new value placed on the dowry as a source of investment capital. As the demands of the

Table 1

Dowry Values 1202-99

	Amount (L)																									
Years	20*	20-29	30-39	40-49	50-59	60-69	70-79	80-89	90-99	100-124	125-149	150-174	175-199	200-249	250-299	300-349	350-399	400-499	500-599	600-699	700-799	800-899	900-999	1000 or More	Total Number Dowries	Total Amount(L) Dowries	Average Amount(L) Dowries+
1202-19	...	3	1	2	2	...	...	...	...	...	...	...	...	...	...	...	...	...	...	...	...	...	...	...	8	277	35
1220-29	2	2	5	4	...	...	2	...	...	...	1	...	1	...	...	...	...	...	...	...	...	...	...	...	17	826	49
1230-39	..	2	2	2	...	2	1	...	...	1	1	...	...	1	...	1	...	1	...	...	...	...	...	...	14	1.539	110
1240-49	2	4	4	1	2	1	3	...	1	2	1	...	...	...	1	1	...	1	...	...	...	1	...	1	26	3,871	149
Total* 1202-49	4	11	12	9	4	3	6	...	1	3	3	...	1	1	1	2	...	2	...	...	...	1	...	1	65	6,513	100
1280-89	1	2	...	1	4	3	3	1	1	3	1	...	...	...	2	...	...	...	1	...	1	...	...	2	26	4,986	191
1290-99	...	1	2	1	1	3	3	2	2	6	2	2	1	1	3	1	1	3	1	...	...	...	1	2	39	8,385	215
Total** 1280-99	1	3	2	2	5	6	6	3	3	9	3	2	1	1	5	1	1	3	2	...	1	...	1	4	65	13,371	205

* Dowry amounts of up to L20.

\+ Rounded to nearest whole number.

* Source: ASS, Archivio Generale dei Contratti; Convento di S. Agostino di Siena; Monastero delle Trafisse; Monte Oliveto Maggiore; Riformagioni; Spedale di Santa Maria della Scala.

** Source: ASS, Archivio Generale dei Contratti.

economy for capital increased, Sienese men may have sought more through marriage exchange, pushing the spiral upwards.

Of course, larger dowries paid to husbands meant larger dowries returned to widows. This point undoubtedly was not lost on Sienese men, who not only had to pay out their daughters' dowries but, as heirs to patrimonies, also had to extract dowry portions from their inheritances to pay off widows. The desire to avoid the disruption this could cause business firms and investments may explain why some husbands' wills offered their wives financial incentives not to seek the return of their dowries.[49] Heirs' refusals to return dowries drove some women to court.[50] It is possible, then, that chronic complaints in the Renaissance period about the increasing costs of dowering women may reflect the real dislocations that the dowry system caused the new economic order. Moreover, by the late thirteenth century, Sienese men realized that women sometimes used the increasing amount of capital contained in their dowries in ways that conflicted with the interests of Siena's patriarchal and patrilineal order.

Husbands never totally controlled their wives' dowries as they did their other property. The law sought to ensure that men would not force their wives to turn over their dowries outright[51] and a husband was prohibited from using the dowry, or a portion of his property obligated for the restitution of a dowry, to pay his debts.[52] Creditors could not demand payment of debts if it could be shown that the property or money they sought was obligated for the restitution of a woman's dowry.[53]

A wife, because of her ultimate ownership of the dowry, might well have had a keen interest in the way her husband conducted his affairs. If a wife believed that her husband was administering her dowry so badly, or was so inept in the management of his business affairs that the eventual restoration of the dowry was endangered, she could demand that it be returned to her immediately. Some wives went to court with this request because their husbands were "on the road to bankruptcy."[54]

Of course, except in extreme or unusual circumstances, a husband had legal and effective control of the dowry until he died.[55] But wives still recognized and acted on their rights as the dowries' owners. Numerous notarial contracts show women selling or ceding the mortgages they held on their husbands' property as creditors for the value of their dowries.[56] Married women also gave away their dowries (or more precisely, their future rights to them) as gifts to individuals and religious institutions and as bequests in wills.[57]

The women who took these actions obviously expected to have their dowries restored someday; indeed the chance that a woman would be widowed and legally entitled to the return of her dowry was good, since it appears that Sienese women, like other urban Italian women, usually married much older men.[58] The *donatione* contracts offer clues to the age difference between spouses, although there is no explicit statement of the ages of the bride or the groom in the dowry or *donatione* contracts or anywhere else. Most *donatione* agreements were made by the groom himself, without the consent of male relatives, indicating that he was at least twenty-five years old, the age of full majority for contractual purposes.[59] Dowry contracts, which were made by the fathers or other relatives of the bride, offer no clues to the women's ages. But the sources which recorded engagement ceremonies do not mention the consent of the brides, which would have been required if she were over fourteen,[60] suggesting, since marriages generally occurred at least several months or a year after the property settlements, that women were probably over fourteen by the time they married. Thus the typical age difference between spouses appears to have been at least eleven years. Further evidence from testaments indicates that wives generally outlived their husbands: in a group of twenty-five testaments drawn between 1283 and 1307, most of which appear to have been written in expectation of imminent death (the testators used the terms *egro* or *egra corpore*), three-quarters of the men making deathbed testaments were married, but only one-quarter of women at the end of their lives still had living husbands (see table 2).

Widowhood, then, was a reasonable expectation for Sienese women, and as widows, most women first came into full possession of the major portion of their capital. The death of a husband, then, generally signalled the birth of a woman's economic autonomy. Some women, either by choice or force of circumstances, may not have taken advantage of their opportunities, but many did retrieve their property from their husbands' estates and established for themselves a measure of economic independence.[61] The way they exercised it in the thirteenth century is the key to understanding the process that brought about the alteration in women's rights and status by the next century.

As we have already seen, Sienese women, married and not mar-

Table 2

Testamentary Bequest Patterns, 1283-1307

Beneficiaries	Total Bequests(N)	Men* Bequests(N)	Men* Testators(N)	Women** Bequests(N)	Women** Testators(N)
Total	193	138	13	55	12
Male	106	87	11	19	9
Female	87	51	13	36	11
Marital Family:					
Total	41	18	9	23	9
Male	14	6	2	8	5
Husband	2	...	...	2	2
Son	12	6	2	6	4
Grandson	0	0	0	0	0
Female	27	12	8	15	5
Wife	7	7	7	...	...
Daughter	17	5	2	12	5
Granddaughter	3	0	0	3	2
Natal Family:					
Total	25	17	9	8	3
Male	13	11	6	2	2
Brother	9	8	5	1	1
Father	0	0	0	0	0
Nephew	4	3	3	1	1
Female	12	6	4	6	3
Sister	9	4	3	5	3
Mother	3	2	2	1	1
Niece	0	0	0	0	0
Others'					
Total	127''	103''	7	24	7
Male	79	70	7	9	6
Female	48	33	6	15	7
Residual:					
Total+	17	9	9	8	8
Male	6	2	...	4	...
Female	8	5	...	3	...
Mixed (M&F)	3	2	...	1	...

Source: ASS, Archivio Generale dei Contratti.

* Ten married, three unmarried.

** Five married, five widowed, two unmarried.

' Individuals not identified as testator's relative.

'' Forty bequests made by one testator.

\+ In addition, one bequest to "the poor."

ried, took advantage of the new commercial opportunities of the thirteenth century. To do this, many may have used wealth not related to their dowries, such as money or property received as a testamentary bequest or as a gift from a relative or friend. No restrictions were placed on their right to freely use this wealth during their adult lives.[62] Also, as has been noted, married women could exercise a measure of control over the disposition of their dowries while their husbands lived. Thus, the economic activities of some widows were similar to those they had undertaken when single or married. The difference was that widows had more capital and less male interference.

The extent of women's independence during any part of the medieval or early modern period is difficult to judge. It has been suggested that one way to measure women's autonomy might be to examine the degree to which they engaged in economic activities with other women, without reference to men.[63] Evidence shows that Sienese women in the thirteenth century bought and sold property jointly or to one another and lent each other money,[64] but these actions still do not tell us how women perceived their economic interests and whether they saw them as different from men's. More significant for this purpose is the evidence that women used the property they inherited and accumulated for the benefit of other women. There are numerous examples of women—married and widowed—giving money or property to other women, especially their daughters and sisters, but also to women who do not appear to be relatives.[65] Although women made similar gifts to men,[66] the gifts given by women to women reflect what might be called a "feminist" orientation—a desire to provide for other women and a consciousness of women's special needs and the restrictions imposed on them by law and custom. This is most clearly seen in women's last wills and testaments.

Unfortunately, few men's and even fewer women's wills survive from the early part of the thirteenth century.[69] Although the number increases after 1250, it still remains extremely small compared with other kinds of documentation. Yet a comparison (summarized in table 2) of men's and women's wills written in the last part of the thirteenth and early fourteenth centuries reveals some startling differences in the ways men and women disposed of their property.[68]

The testaments in table 2 were drawn between 1283 and 1307, a time when women had more property to dispose of than they had earlier in the century, primarily because of increased dowries, and, in some cases, profits from commercial and real estate investments. The most striking pattern that emerges from a comparison of the bequests made by women and men is that, overwhelmingly, women left their property to other women while men left theirs to other men. While 63 percent of men's bequests were to males, only 37 percent were made to females. The women made only 35 percent of their bequests to males and 65 percent to females, almost the exact reverse ratio. A closer scrutiny of the bequests made to various categories of heirs—marital and natal relatives and unrelated individuals (or at least persons with no specified relationship)—yields similar results. In most of the categories men favored men and women favored women as their heirs.[69]

Perhaps the most significant differences can be found in the bequests made to children and grandchildren. While men made an almost equal number to sons and daughters, women made the majority of their bequests to daughters and granddaughters, favoring female descendants over male by a ratio to five to two. Almost 75 percent of all the bequests made to female descendants were made by women.

Many more men than women made bequests to their natal kin (brothers, sisters, and nephews) and the men heavily favored males. In fact, the men favored male heirs by a ratio of almost two to one, while women favored females by three to two. This pattern reinforces the impression given by the bequests to children that men, but not women, were concerned with preserving property in the male line.[70]

The bequests to apparently unrelated persons (called "others" in table 2) also confirm the pattern of women favoring women and men, men. Sixty-eight percent of men's bequests were to men and 32 percent were to women, while 63 percent of women's bequests were to women and only 37 percent to men. The large number and the nature of bequests in this category indicate that friendship and personal affection were important considerations to the people making these wills and that members of each sex had stronger feelings toward friends of their own sex.

Another important series of bequests was those to "residual heirs," the persons who were to inherit the remainder of the testators' property. Residual heirs included wives, a husband, a mother, brothers, a nephew, and even a sister-in-law. While both men and women named sons as residual heirs, no man named a daughter. In every case in which a daughter was bequeathed the remainder of all the goods in an estate, it was done by her mother.

One explanation for fathers' relative neglect of their daughters in favor of sons and other male relatives is that daughters had already received their share of the patrimony in the form of their dowries. But in middle- and upper-class families, sons were very likely partners in their fathers' business firms, and might well have come into possession of large shares of the patrimony through that association. So might have brothers and nephews, who were often business associates.[71] When writing their wills testators could make additional bequests to any individual they chose. Men usually chose other men as their beneficiaries, particularly men of their patrilineage. Women, on the other hand, diverted property away from male to female family members and friends, capital which, if they had not made testaments, would have passed by law to their sons or other male relatives.

The women's testaments reveal another important pattern of preferences. Widows, who generally had the most property and independence, favored female relatives over males to an even greater degree than did married women (see table 3). Quite possibly, by the time a widow made her will, her sons and other male relatives had been provided for by other men, while her daughters and female relations had not fared so well: the widows bequests may have been attempts to remedy that situation.

Thus, when women made their wills they were specifically taking the opportunity to express their personal wishes for the disposition of their property—and these differed significantly from men's. The more property a woman had—and, generally, she would have more in widowhood—the more the expression of those preferences differed from men's. Furthermore, women's choices for their beneficiaries were not those men whom the authorities of the Commune would have recognized as their rightful heirs had they died intestate.

Thus, by the end of the thirteenth century, just at the time that middle- and upper-class women were accumulating increasing amounts of capital, women's economic independence came under attack. During the latter part of the century, a statutory reaction to women's control over their wealth began. The Commune of Siena enacted a series of laws which placed progressively more severe restrictions on women's ability to use and dispose of their property. Although the stated purpose of the laws was to "protect the rights of children" to inherit their mothers' property, their aim, in fact, was to ensure that it passed to male heirs. For example, the law code of 1262 included a statute which forbade any woman, "married or not," who had children, from making a testament, gift, sale, or other alienation of her dotal property which would deprive her surviving children of their rightful inheritance when she died. She could freely dispose of only one-quarter.[72] Of course, if a woman

Table 3

Testamentary Bequest Patterns of
Married and Widowed Women, 1283-1307

Beneficiaries	Total Bequests(N)	Married Women Bequests(N)	Married Women Testators(N)	Widows Bequests(N)	Widows Testators(N)
Total	48	24	5	24	5
Male	16	11	5	5	3
Female	32	13	4	19	5
Marital Family:					
Total	23	10	5	13	4
Male	8	6	4	2	1
Husband	2	2	2	...	...
Son	6	4	3	2	1
Grandson	0	0	0	0	0
Female	15	4	2	11	3
Daughter	12	4	2	8	3
Granddaughter	3	0	0	3	2
Natal Family:					
Total	4	3	1	1	1
Male	1	1	1	0	0
Brother	1	1	1	0	0
Father	0	0	0	0	0
Nephew	0	0	0	0	0
Female	3	2	1	1	1
Sister	3	2	1	1	1
Mother	0	0	0	0	0
Niece	0	0	0	0	0
Others*:					
Total	21	11	3	10	3
Male	8	5	3	3	2
Female	13	6	3	7	2
Residual:					
Total	7	4	4	3	3
Male	3	2	2	1	1
Female	3	1	1	2	2
Mixed (M&F)	1	1	1	0	0

Source: ASS, Archivio Generale dei Contratti.

* Individuals not identified as relatives.

did not leave a will, and most did not, her dowered daughters could not share in the inheritance with their brothers, so the rights of the children actually meant the rights of sons. A statute of 1283 went even further, invalidating any contract made by a woman even before her marriage which would threaten the rights of any children she might have subsequently to inherit her dowry. The law specified loans, sales, and gifts, as well as any other contract made with a woman's male relatives, any other man, or "other person."[73] Although probably intended to prevent a woman's relatives from attempting to recover her dowry by making a contractual arrangement with her, this statute allowed for the possibility that children born years after a contract had been made could claim that it was prejudicial to their rights and have it voided. This statute also upheld the financial interests of husbands at the expense of wives' independence. It increased the portion of a childless wife's dowry that a husband could retain on her death from one-third to one-half[74] (the other half would return to her father). Since that half of the dowry was specifically reserved for her husband, a childless woman was prohibited from freely disposing of it during her lifetime. To reinforce men's rights, another law forbade any married woman from making sales, gifts, or any other obligation of her dowry without the consent of her husband.[75] If enforced, these statutes would have effectively barred women from all independent real estate and commercial activities, since no rational person of either sex would have entered into a contractual arrangement with a woman at any time during her life.

The evidence of notarial documents shows that, at least in the thirteenth and early fourteenth centuries, these statutes did not have that drastic effect. Yet, this legislation marks a critical turning point in the history of Sienese women. While these laws did not reflect the economic roles women actually played in this period, they attempted to define what those roles should be in the future. This legislation sought to eliminate the gains women had made during the late medieval period and substantially reduce their economic influence and legal and social independence.

Thus, the transformation of the Sienese economy, which initially brought expanded opportunities for women, resulted in the restriction of women's options as men moved to reserve capital and capital investment for themselves. Although women's nominal wealth had increased, their legal rights to control it had diminished. These changes augured poorly for the future, since wealth over which one has control becomes qualitatively different from wealth over which one does not. By the fourteenth century, women's wealth was defined as different from men's. It was not to be the wealth which commercial society valued and upon which the economy depended. That wealth was to belong to, and be controlled by, men.

REFERENCES

This article was originally written at the suggestion of Joan Kelly, whose guidance and comments were, as always, invaluable. I wish to thank Heath Dillard and Alice Miller for their aid and patience in the preparation of this version.

1. Joan Kelly-Gadol, "Did Women have a Renaissance?" in *Becoming Visible,* ed. R. Bridenthal and C. Koonz (Boston, 1977): 139-64; also see her article "The Social Relation of the Sexes: Methodological Implications of Women's History," *Signs: Journal of Women in Culture and Society* 1, no. 4 (Summer 1976): 809-23.

2. See Dina Bizzarri, "Introduction," to *Imbreviature notarile,* vol. 1, *Liber imbreviature Appuliesis notarii Communis Senarum MCCXXI-MCCXXIII, ed. Dina Bizzarri (Siena, 1934; reprint ed., Turin, 1970),* lxii-xi (hereafter Bizzarri, *Imbreviature notarile,* vols. 1 or 2, followed by the number of the document); and Mario Chiaudano, "Introduction," to vol. 2, *Liber imbreviature Ildibrandini notarii MCCXVII-MCCXXIX* (Siena, 1938; reprint ed., Turin, 1970), lxxxix-cxi (hereafter Chiaudano). The edited notarial documents contained in these two volumes will be cited as *Imbreviature notarile,* vols. 1 or 2, followed by the number of the document.

3. See Chiaudano, xcvii, lc, cx-cxi.

4. Chiaudano, li; Bizzarri, *Imbreviature* introduction, xxxciiiff. For the effects of Roman and Germanic law on women see Franco Ercole, "L'istituto dotale nella practica e nella legislazione statuaria dell'Italia superiore," *Rivista italiana per le scienze giuridiche* 45 (1908): 191-302; 46 (1910): 167-257 (hereafter Ercole, 1 or 2), and idem, "Vicende storiche della dote romana nella practica medievale dell'Italia superiore," *Archivio giuridico* 80 (1908): 393-490 and 81 (1908): 34-148; A. Pertile, *Storia del diritto italiano,* 2d ed. 3 (Turin, 1894), 76-79, 232-44; Francesco Brandileone, "Studi preliminari sullo svolgimento storico dei rapporti patrimoniale fra coniugi in Italia," in *Scritti di storia del diritto privato italiano* 1 (Bologna, 1931), 229-319; Katherine Drew, *The Lombard Laws* (Philadelphia, 1973).

5. For women's contractual rights see Bizzarri, *Imbreviature* introduction, xxxviii, and idem, *Il diritto privato nelle fonte senese del secolo XIII,* 2 vols. (Siena, 1921), 1:54 (hereafter *Diritto privato*). Most laws relating to women's property rights are found in *Il constituto del Comune di Siena dell'anno 1262,* ed. Lodovico Zdekauer (Milan, 1897), and *Il costituto del Comune di Siena volgarizzatto nel 1309-10,* 2 vols. ed. A. Lisini (Siena, 1903) (hereafter *Const. 1262* and *Const. 1309-10),* esp. Dist. II of *Const. 1262* and Dist. II and V of *Const. 1309-10.*

6. Archivio di Stato di Siena, (hereafter ASS) Diplomatico, *Archivio Generale dei Contratti,* 1224, November 2; 1304, December 7 (hereafter *AG*); ASS, *Spedale di Santa Maria della Scala,* 1229, August 12 (hereafter *Spedale*). See also ASS, Ospedale di Santa Maria della Scala, *Contratti e Protocolli,* 71.

7. *Imbreviature notarile,* vol. 2, no. 264; *AG,* 1255, January 21.

8. *AG,* 1255, January 7.

9. *Imbreviature notarile,* vol. 1, no. 496; In 1223, two men paid Bonafemina fifty lire, which they and their business partners owed her "*pro cambio sterlingarum.*"

10. See Chiaudano, lxxiv; and Bizzarri, *Imbreviature* introduction, xli.

11. E.g., see *Imbreviature notarile,* vol. 2, no. 66; *AG,* 1304, May (no day).

12. Bizzarri considers the development and use of the surety instrument as one of the major signs of Siena's "precocious" commercial development. *Imbreviature,* introduction, lxiii.

13. *Imbreviature notarile,* vol. 1, no. 60; vol. 2, no. 226.

14. *Imbreviature notarile,* vols. 1 and 2.

15. It should be noted that real estate transactions may be underrepresented in these notebooks since property located in the suburbs or *contado* might have been recorded by notaries in those areas.

16. Coincidentally, perhaps, table 1 shows that dowries also ranged from 20 *soldi* to just under £ 200 in the 1220s. See the discussion of dowry amounts below.

17. Fourteen out of sixteen contracts in 1221-23, four out of five in 1227-29.

18. *Const. 1262,* Dist. II, r. xxxiv, xxxvii, xxxix, xl; *Const. 1309-10,* Dist. II, r. xliii, xlix, li-iii. See also Bizzarri, *Diritto privato,* 1:65; and Ercole, 1: 289-91 for the principles upon which Sienese legislation was based.

19. *Const. 1262,* Dist. II, r. xxxvii.

20. Ibid., r. xxxviii; *Const. 1309-10,* Dist. II, r. xlii, xlv, liii.

21. *Const. 1262,* Dist. II, r. xxxiv, xl; *Const. 1309-10,* Dist. II, r. xlii, xlv.

22. See Ercole, 1: 212; and Diane Owen Hughes' article in this volume, "From Brideprice to Dowry in Mediterranean Europe," pp. 32-33. See also J. Goody and S.J. Tambiah, *Bridewealth and dowry* (Cambridge, 1973).

23. The first instance of a Roman dowry was 1144, see Chiaudano, 1. Sienese marriage customs have been said to "correspond perfectly" to Roman principles (Bizzarri, *Imbreviature* introduction, xxxviii). For a discussion of the change from Germanic brideprice to dowry, see Diane Owen Hughes' article in this volume. For marriage exchange see Ercole, 1 and 2; and idem, "Vicende storiche"; Brandileone, "Studi preliminari"; and idem, *Sulla storia e natura della "donatione propter nuptias"* (Bologna, 1892); Bizzarri, *Diritto privato.* See below for a discussion of the *donatione propter nuptias* in Siena.

24. Normally death, but marriage could also be terminated by divorce or when one spouse entered a religious order. See Ercole, 2: 222-23.

25. *Const. 1262,* Dist. II, r. xix.

26. Ibid., r. lxvi-iii.

27. Ibid., r. xxx, xxxv; *Const. 1309-10,* Dist. II, r. xl, xliv, xlvii.

28. *Const. 1262,* Dist. II, r. xxx, xxxv.

29. Prior to the middle of the century a separate Curia Mulierum had jurisdiction over most cases involving women. This court ceased to function during the first part of the century and most matters concerning women were transferred to the other judges of the Commune. Questions involving dowry were placed under the Curia del Placito. See Bizzarri, *Diritto privato,* 1:53; Chiaudano, xxxi.

30. E.g., Ospedale di Santa Maria della Scala, *Contratti e Protocolli,* no. 71 contains complete copies of twenty-six men's testaments drawn between 1238 and 1279. Only five contain bequests to daughters. For examples of bequests by fathers and other male relatives see *AG,* 1249, January 4; 1305, December 10; ASS, Diplomatico, *Convento di San Agostino,* 1231, November 21, (hereafter *Agostino*); *Il Caleffo Vecchio del Comune di Siena,* 3 vols., ed. G. Cecchini (Siena, 1931-40), esp. nos. 410, 414.

31. *AG,* 1249, September 19; ASS, Diplomatico, *Riformagioni,* 1246, November 17.

32. *AG,* 1297, August 21.

33. See e.g., *Agostino,* 1240, May 4; *AG,* 1232, October 30; 1298, April 5; 1294, April 17.

34. See e.g., *AG,* 1226, March 9.

35. See ibid., 1249, September 19.

36. See, e.g., ASS. *Guida-Inventario,* (Siena, 1953) 1:267.

37. See esp. Ercole, 1: 197.

38. In this early stage of commercial capitalism, Siena lacked most modern financial instruments, so the dowry may well have been an important source of investment capital. See Bizzarri, *Imbreviature,* introduction, xli; Chiaudano, lxxiv.

39. A particularly good source of these contracts is the *AG.* See also A. Lisini, *Inventario delle pergamene conservate nel diplomatico dall'anno 736 all'anno 1250* (Siena, 1903).

40. See, e.g., *Spedale,* 1249, August 8; *Agostino,* 1243, September 17. The Commune required that a husband pay a tax on the dowry he received, whether it was given in coins, properties, or "things and rights and credit instruments." William M. Bowsky, *The Finance of the Commune of Siena* (Oxford, 1970), 153.

41. See Hughes, "From Brideprice to Dowry."

42. Of the 130 contracts in table 1, only 22 confer a dowry.

43. In the *donatione* contracts the groom guaranteed that the dowry would be restored to his wife "within the time prescribed by law," which was one year. See *Const. 1262,* Dist. II,

r. xxx. He then pledged this property to cover the obligation, sometimes stipulating that, if necessary, all his property was pledged for that purpose. See, e.g., *Imbreviature notarile,* vol. 1, no. 185; vol. 2, no. 313. For the nature of the *donatione propter nuptias* see Chiaudano, lvii-iii; Brandileone, *Sulla storia e natura della "donatione propter nuptias";* P. Vaccari, *Scritti di storia del diritto privato* (Padua, 1956), 83-102; Bizzarri, *Diritto privato.* See also Hughes, "From Brideprice to Dowry."

44. E.g., *AG,* 1233, January 21, where a brother settles a debt of sixteen lire for his sister's dowry by giving his brother-in-law a piece of land.

45. Of the sixty-five contracts drawn between 1200 and 1249 in table 1 only three mention property without a cash value (*inextimata*). Of the sixty-five drawn between 1280 and 1299, only two do so.

46. In fact, the Commune specifically forbade women from inheriting one type of real estate with considerable symbolic significance: "towers" or "palaces attached to towers." The symbols and foci of activity of urban "consortial" families, towers represented family solidarity, power, and pride in lineage. See *Const. 1262,* Dist. II, r. xxxviii; *Const. 1309-10,* Dist. II, r. lii; and see Daniel Waley, *The Italian City-Republic* (New York, 1969), 170-78. J. Kirshner and A. Molho have noted that in Florence, "cash and liquid assets predominated in dotal settlements" in order that real property "whenever possible did not travel with the wife to her husband and his family but remained with her father, brothers, and male kin." ("The Dowry Fund and the Marriage Market in Early Quattrocento Florence," *Journal of Modern History* 50 [September 1978]: 435-36).

47. Ercole, 1: 280-84; see Stanley Chojnacki, "Dowries and Kinsmen in Early Renaissance Venice," *Journal of Interdisciplinary History* 5 (Spring 1975): 272-73.

48. David Herlihy, "Life Expectancies for Women in Medieval Society," In Rosemarie Thee Morewedge, ed. *The Role of Women in the Middle Ages* (Albany, N.Y., 1975), 12; reprinted in David Herlihy, *The Social History of Italy and Western Europe, 700-1500* (London, 1978). See also idem, "The Medieval Marriage Market," *Medieval and Renaissance Studies* 6 (1976) 3-21; reprinted in David Herlihy, *The Social History of Italy and Western Europe, 700-1500* (London, 1978). But see Hughes, "From Brideprice to Dowry," p. 40 for a criticism of his method.

49. See the wills cited in note 31.

50. *AG,* 1249, January 18; 1232, December 31.

51. See note 25.

52. *Const. 1262,* Dist. II, r. lxvi

53. Ibid., r. lxvi, lxvii, lxix; *Const. 1309-10,* Dist. II, r. lxxxv-ix. These provisions, could, of course, be used by less scrupulous men to their own advantages. Probably recognizing this possibility, the law sought to limit the instances where men would try to avoid paying their debts by insisting that if a husband and his wife refused to pay a debt, claiming such payment would have to be made out of dotal property, the husband's property could be sold off, the wife paid her dowry, and the remainder used to pay off the husband's creditors. Another statute, *Const. 1262,* Dist. II, r. lxx, specifically forbade a husband from fraudulently turning over property to his wife as repayment of her dowry in order to avoid his creditors.

To ensure that property involved in a sale or transfer would not at a later time be claimed to be under obligation for a dowry, husbands had their wives make formal renunciations of all present and future rights to that property in the contract of sale or transfer. See, e.g., *Imbreviature notarile,* vol. 2, no. 48.

54. See, e.g., *AG,* 1246, December (no day); 1249, May 13; 1254, December 9; 1280, December 13. See also Lodovico Zdekauer, *La vita privata senese nel dugento* (Siena, 1896; reprint ed., Bologna, 1967), 96.

55. A woman could also have her dowry restored if she left her husband's house because she was "gravely offended" by him or his relatives. *Const. 1262,* Dist. II, r. xxx.

56. See, e.g., *Spedale,* 1225, May 6.

57. E.g., *AG,* 1302, July 24; see also tables 1 and 2.

58. David Herlihy has written extensively on this topic; see esp. "The Medieval Mar-

riage Market," 18-19. See also "Deaths, Marriages, Births and the Tuscan Economy (ca. 1300-1500)," in *Population Patterns in the Past,* ed. Ronald Demos Lee (New York, 1977) 143-52; "The Tuscan Town in the Quattrocento: A Demographic Profile," *Medievalia et Humanistica* n.s. 1 (1970): 92; "Marriage at Pistoia in the Fifteenth Century," *Bulletino Storico Pistoiese* 3d. ser., 7 (1972): 3-21 (all are reprinted in David Herlihy, *Cities and Society in Medieval Italy* [London, 1980]).

59. 108 of the 130 contracts in table 1 were made by grooms; see *Const. 1262,* Dist. II, r. xcviii, cv, cxiv.

60. Bizzarri, *Diritto privato,* 2:8; *AG,* 1301, June 28; 1301, February 11.

61. See esp. *AG,* 1295, May 11, and *Spedale,* 1244, April 16 for restitution by a son; *AG,* 1244, March 31 for restitution by a guardian in the name of minor children; and 1244, February 12 for restitution by the brothers of the deceased.

62. Ercole, 1: 201

63. Kathleen Casey, "Female Virtù in Italy's Rural Renaissance" (paper presented at the Berkshire Conference on the History of Women, Cambridge, Mass., October, 1974).

64. See ASS, Diplomatico, *Convento di San Francesco di Siena,* 1232, November 11, and *Imbreviature notarile,* vols. 1 and 2.

65. *Imbreviature notarile,* vol. 1, no. 89; *AG,* 1292, October 10; 1293, April 30; 1302, December 10.

66. E.g., *AG,* 1296, November 1.

67. *Imbreviature notarile,* vols. 1 and 2 contain only four wills each, two men's and two women's. See vol. 1, nos. 393, 437; vol. 2, nos. 177, 299.

68. In *AG,* MS B87, the same body of documents where the late thirteenth century dowries in table 1 are found, there are twelve complete, extant women's wills for the years 1280-1307, not many, but a large number in comparison to earlier years. There are also increased references to women's testaments which are no longer preserved (see, e.g., *AG,* 1293, December 4). For an informative use of women's testaments in Venice see Chojnacki, "Dowries and Kinsmen," esp., 586.

69. If bequests to spouses are deducted from the totals, men's bequests to males constitute a much larger proportion of their bequests.

70. For example, in bequests to siblings, sisters were the largest group in women's bequests, brothers in men's. Only one woman made a bequest to a brother; the only woman's bequest to a nephew was to her sister's son.

71. Testaments were merely incomplete, discrete lists of properties and beneficiaries. The remainder of the testator's property may have been disposed of at other times in other ways. See Chiaudano, lix and notes 65 and 66 above, for women's gifts to living persons.

72. *Const. 1262,* Dist. II, r. xxxi.

73. *Const. 1309-10,* Dist. II, r. xxviii. The 1309-10 code was based on a Latin text of 1296. There had been several revisions of the code after 1262, incorporating changes in the law. The compilation of 1309-10 remained in force until 1337. See Lisini, introduction, *Const. 1309-10,* iv.

74. *Const. 1262,* Dist. II, r. xxxvi had allowed a husband to retain one-third.

75. *Const. 1309-10,* Dist. II, r. xxx

Trousseau as Treasure: Some Contradictions of Late Nineteenth-Century Change in Sicily

Jane Schneider

INTRODUCTION

On the eve of her wedding, a Sicilian bride displays her trousseau (called *corredo),* spreading its contents out on bed, chairs, and tables for invited guests to see. Today, the principal items of a trousseau are money plus commercially available household goods—tablewear and linens, furniture, and small appliances. Until two or three decades ago, however, ensembles known as "beds" (*letti*) predominated. A bed referred not to the piece of furniture, but to the bed coverings: two sheets, four pillowcases, a bedspread, and lingerie for the bride. Indeed, each bed was a cluster of whitewear (*biancheria*) that could include table cloths, napkins, towels, doilies, pillowcases, and intimate apparel, as well as sheets.

Most pieces of whitewear were hand embroidered or trimmed with handmade lace, each containing many women-hours of work. So great was women's commitment to trousseau preparation and to the needle arts in general, that other kinds of work in agriculture and industry were precluded, even when the opportunity for such work was there. Some observers of Mediterranean societies—most recently John Davis—suggest that cultural patterns making female labor unavailable for income-producing activities have impeded agrarian transformation and economic development in the area.[1] If this is a correct perception, then Sicily is a striking example.

Since the late nineteenth century, Sicily has specialized in the export of migrant workers, first to the Americas, subsequently to northern Europe. This exodus, constant except for a hiatus during and between the two world wars, and serious enough to have been

"Trousseau as Treasure: Some Contradictions of Late Nineteenth-Century Change in Sicily," by Jane Schneider is taken from *Beyond the Myths of Culture,* Eric Ross, editor, Academic Press, 1980

called "Italy's hemorrhage," was a consequence of the island's failure to produce alternative exports for world markets. Perhaps contributions of female labor could have made a difference to the cost-competitiveness of agricultural or industrial commodities and thus stemmed the tide of out-migration. Historical evidence suggests, however, that embroidered beds became the staple of nonaristocratic trousseau in Sicily just as the mass migrations got underway.

This chapter poses the question: "What happened in the late nineteenth century which led ordinary women to take up needlework on a scale before unknown?" Data are from several sources. In a recent field trip, Peter Schneider and I obtained information from the vital registers of Villamaura, the pseudonym for a rural town of about 7500 population, where we also conducted research in the 1960s.[2] This information provides the basis for a family reconstitution study which will compare the reproductive patterns of marriage cohorts (we sampled all marriages for 1850-1851, 1860-1861, 1870-1871, 1880-1881, 1890, 1899, 1910, and 1920) and by occupational group. (Villamaura, like most Sicilian settlements, is internally stratified; large landowners, professionals, merchants, shopkeepers, artisans, rich, middle, and proletarianized peasants have lived in close proximity for a long time.) Supplementing this demographic record are minutes of town council meetings beginning in 1860, house and land cadasters for the 1870s, lists of trousseau recorded by folklorists and in the archives of the notary public, oral histories, secondary sources, and a range of artifacts that we came upon by asking people to show us old houses, furniture, clothing, photographs, and products of local craftsmanship including embroidery.

In the following pages, I will first describe the marriage exchange system as it existed until a few years ago and then present evidence that embroidered whitewear was not a timeless part of it with roots in an unchanging past. The question "why embroidery" will be broached in three different contexts. The first has to do with class formation and the emulation of elite behavior; the second with symbolic links between embroidery and female purity, an important behavioral code in the Mediterranean. The third interprets evidence that embroidered sheets were wealth objects with significant liquidity in wide spheres of exchange. These three approaches are neither contradictory nor mutually exclusive; they complement and reinforce one another. I think, however, that the third, which conceives of trousseau as treasure, raises new and interesting questions about folk culture.

TROUSSEAU AND SOCIAL REPRODUCTION

A trousseau of "beds," or sheets with whitewear in proportion, is hardly unique to Sicily. Brides all over southern Europe are, or were, similarly endowed at marriage. Ethnographies of this area, moreover, offer relatively consistent estimates of the number of beds or sheets that distinguish rich girls from poor girls. In Pitkin's south Italian study of the 1950s, 6 sheets (plus supporting whitewear) constituted a minimum *corredo.* The majority of brides brought 12; daughters of rich peasants and merchants married with 24; those of lesser landowners with 50; and women whose families owned large estates brought up to 100 sheets.[3] This range is probably similar to that of Pisticci, where Davis (1973) found the minimum to be three "beds" and it matches closely the estimates given to me in Villamaura.[4] In Silverman's Umbrian town, the poorest brides had 10 to 12 sheets, the richest 48 or more.[5]

Trousseaux of whatever quantity represented a considerable expense for the bride's family. From the time she was born, her father and brothers labored to purchase the materials of which a respectable *corredo* was made, this responsibility being formalized in the saying, heard often in Villamaura, "swaddling clothes on the baby girl, whitewear in her hope chest" (*bambine nelle fascie, biancheria nella cascia*). To facilitate the preparation of trousseau brothers delayed their own marriages until their sisters were wed or, for those sisters who did not marry, until they were securely set up in careers of respectable celibacy as nuns, "house nuns," or servants of close kin.

While father and brothers put their earnings into basic *corredo* materials, mother and daughters invested labor in their elaboration, with mother serving as organizer and supervisor, and daughters doing most of the work. Before the age of 7 years, most daughters were skilled at sample stitching, and during their adolescence they became devotees of embroidery, sacrificing hours in the interest of perfection. Compared with other crafts, embroidery and lacework are not so much difficult as they are extremely tedious. Gömül, an expert on Turkish embroidery, says that like "digging a well with a needle," it requires the greatest effort, time, and patience of all the crafts.[6] Nor could the effort be spread throughout the year. Sicilian women rarely embroidered in the summer months, not because they had to work at the harvest but because the heat made their hands sweat: In the winter, days were short, and a craft that fatigued their eyes under the best of conditions became burdensome when done by candlelight or oil lamp. (Rural electrification came to the Sicilian interior in the 1920s.)

The preparation of trousseau was so costly in terms of both money and time, that Sicilians used to say, during Chapman's fieldwork in the late 1920s, that they had "six children, two boys and four burdens," even though they loved their daughters and counted more on their affection than the affection of sons to sustain them in later life. People also told Chapman that the door through which a dead daughter passed is "blessed . . . and the older she is the greater the comfort; if she is single she relieves us from debt; if she is engaged she gives us life; and if she is married she fills the pot."[7] This expression refers to the legal and customary arrangement whereby a wife's property reverted to her natal family (her parents or brothers) if she died before having children of her own.

Of course, women's property could consist of many things, usually transferred to her as dowry at the time of her marriage. Trousseau is only one component of dowry along with land, houses, money, and education. Until the twentieth century, however, and probably until the 1930s, trousseau predominated in the dowries of nonaristocratic Sicilian girls. John Davis argues for Pisticci that this is a reasonable conclusion when the tax registers for land and houses show women owners to be in a small minority. A land cadaster for Villamaura drawn up in 1870 lists 3288 parcels of land of which 161 belonged to women. Of these, widows held 87 and 34 were in the landowning class. Only 12 parcels of land, out of more than 3000, belonged to untitled women and all were extremely small, less than a hectare.

A house cadaster, prepared in 1877 for the 1881 census, suggests that houses sometimes entered dowry. Less than 2500 actual households (for a then population of 9682) appear in that census for Villamaura, but the tax register, making note of all rooms with a doorway to the street, has nearly 4000 entries.[8] Of these, 20 were attributed to women as members of groups of heirs; 250 to widows; and 395 to individual women, a few of whom were spinsters, the great majority married. In contrast to the land cadaster, untitled women were well represented in the latter group, but the group is far too small to conclude that, in the late 1870s, houses were transferred to daughters as a general rule.

Toward the end of the nineteenth century, an increasing number of nonaristocratic families went to the trouble of having their daughters' dowries registered with a notary public, which makes the notary's archive another source of information on dotal property. Of the 68 couples who married in Villamaura in 1880, the families of 20 (or 32%) visited the notary to register dowries, as did families of 18 (26%) of the 68 couples who married in 1890. They were rich peasants, storekeepers, an occasional carter and artisan, 10 peasants,[9] and 3 titled landowners. Most of them gave their daughters tiny parcels of land, which in all but 10 cases measured less than half a hectare, and in all but 2, less than a hectare. Slightly less than half gave small houses, ususally of one or two rooms. As Davis indicates for Pisticci, the value of the *corredo* nearly equalled and in some cases surpassed the value of these token immovables. Similarly, 13 of the registered dowries included money, but in 10 of these, the amount was less than the trousseau's recorded value.

Given the likelihood that unregistered dowries contained no land, houses, or money, the situation for late nineteenth-century Villamaura appears to have approached Silverman's description of Umbria a few years ago: "For most girls the corredo and furniture are the total dowry, but a well-to-do family might also give a daughter money or property at her marriage, as an advance against her share of the family patrimony."[10] How far into the twentieth century trousseau remained the central component of dowry in Sicily is hard to estimate on the basis of data available to me now. In Villamaura, as in Pisticci, landholdings began to fragment after about 1910 and gradually women acquired more of them, but the relationship between these developments is far from clear. It is possible that land divisions mandated by various reform programs increased the number of women owners by putting more of this resource into peasant hands. It is also possible, however, that fathers added more land (and houses) to the dowries of their daughters for reasons not directly related to land reform, with the consequence of accelerating land fragmentation.

There remains the further problem raised by Davis (1973) that in the underdeveloped regions of the Italian south and islands, land was losing its value as a source of agricultural productivity even before it was expropriated from large holders and redistributed, so much so that symbolic reasons for having it increased in proportion to reasons of economic security or gain, making women's ownership somewhat spurious.[11] Perhaps this is why women whom I interviewed in 1977 claimed that, until very recently when education took over, trousseau remained the set-piece of a respectable dowry. One could always marry without land, houses or money, but never without trousseau, and several informants spontaneously recalled exemplary families who had recently sold off land to acquire their daughter's linens.

Further evidence that trousseau was central to marriage exchanges (the counterpart of a groom's promise to support his wife) are the institutions in Sicily (Southern Italy also) of the *minuta* and the *stima.* The *minuta,* no longer practiced, took place when the families of a newly engaged couple brought in a literate person, mutually agreed upon, to enumerate the goods that each was committing to the eventual new household. More important was the *stima (la vagghiata dell robba, or vagghiu,* in dialect), which occurred on the eve of the wedding, when the bride's family hired a specialized *stimatrice (vagghiatura)* to examine each article of assembled trousseau and price it. Usually a woman knowledgeable about textiles, the *stimatrice* assigned and recorded values in lire or onze, the currency of earlier regimes.[12]

Both the *minuta* and *stima* resulted in formal, written contracts, as they had for aristocratic families in earlier centuries.[13] Some of these contracts were notarized, but even when they were not, people kept the papers on which they were written, thereby protecting the claims of natal kin should they die without heirs. In a way the *stima* was the pivotal event of a Sicilian marriage. Attended by witnesses as well as the close relatives of the couple, it was an occasion not only for proud display, but sometimes for quarreling, as the bride's family pressed for high estimates, which the groom's family felt were a disadvantage to them, whether in balancing her wealth with land, or in the event it should have to be returned. Because the groom's family gained in status from a high valuation, however, this conflict of interests was usually overcome; then, in a joyous ritual, friends and relatives of the bride carried her handiwork, piece by piece, to the house where she would take up residence, one of them staying to act as guardian during the night.[14]

STATUS EMULATION, CLASS FORMATION, AND THE SPREAD OF NEEDLEWORK

Trousseau was a central, and for many families the only, component of dowry throughout the nineteenth and well into the twentieth century, but its content seems to have changed in the course of this period. In 1808, Paolo Balsamo, a Sicilian propagandist for agrarian reform in the style of Arthur Young (whom he knew), wrote a memorandum urging his countrymen to cultivate linen despite the obstacles that an arid environment placed in the way of this endeavor. His argument was that "shirts, underwear, sheets, table cloths, napkins, towels and swaddling bands. . .bring to clothing and furniture that tidiness which enhances and adorns the civilized life."[15] The tone of his plea suggests that these articles were not yet in wide use among the peasants of his day, even though limited amounts of hemp (*canapa*) were cultivated, and hemp is a good, if coarse, substitute for linen.

In urging the acceptance of more "linens," Balsamo recognized that they were not necessities, but neither were they luxuries, he argued. He would have appreciated the term "decencies," which an English economic historian recently coined for just such things as sheets and underwear.[16] In contrast, the same memorandum claimed that "lace and similar exquisite and fine work . . . serve to content the insatiable desire for appearances, pomp and luxury, among the rich and the great."[17] From this we can assume that ornamented "decencies" were at that time largely enjoyed by Sicily's landowning aristocracy and court.

That ornamentation of whitewear in the form of embroidery and lace was a luxury that few could afford in the early nineteenth century is also documented by the content of the trousseaux. Salvatore Salmone-Marino, a folklorist of the late 1800s, collected a few contracts of *minuta* dating back to 1810 and in none of them is there any reference to embroidery, except for minimal decorations on handkerchiefs and swaddling cloths for infants.[18] The same lack of attention to embroidery characterizes the notarized trousseaux which Pitrè found for 1847 and 1855, both for modest peasant families.[19] Nevertheless, Pitrè's examples, and Salomone-Marino's too, include several articles of bed-, table-, and underwear.

Working back from the present, oral histories collected in Villamaura in 1977, supplemented by a look at artifacts, give the impression that all but the poorest women married with richly embroidered "beds" from the turn of the century and probably a decade or two earlier. How to date the appearance of this custom is problematic, given that only a minority of families went to the trouble and expense of notarizing dowry before 1900. Nevertheless, many hints exist in the data on women's changing round of chores to be discussed in the following. For the moment, I think it is safe to assume that we are talking about a transition that occurred in the late 1800s, although at different rates for different occupational groups and different towns.

One way of characterizing, and perhaps understanding, the elaboration of embroidery in folk culture is to trace its diffusion through a process of status emulation similar to the one outlined in Veblen's study of the leisure class. An important reason why, in earlier centuries, only noble women were the owners of richly decorated linens is that they were freed by slaves, servants, and other dependents from many household tasks, leaving them with time to embroider. One is reminded that even in New England, "the possession of a good piece of old crewel work, done in the country, is as strong a proof of respectable ancestry as a patent of nobility, since no one in the busy early colonial days had time for such work save those whose abundant leisure was secured by ample means and liberal surroundings".[20]

In addition to offering a marker of leisure status, embroideries and lacework conferred prestige by removing the materials to which they were applied several more steps from their natural state as fibers, and from the natural, bodily functions which they were intended to transform. Richard and Sally Price witnessed an extreme example of this in a small Spanish village in 1964 where the trousseau of a prosperous peasant girl included six monogrammed sanitary napkins.[21] Often embroidered whitewear was so totally separated from anything resembling nature that it was not even used. Indeed, in contrast to the textile labors of women in the lower classes, embroidery and lacework produced finery that was largely for entertainment, gift-giving and display, and for eventual transfer to daughters as heirlooms.[22] Whether used or not, however, periodic laundering and sun-bleaching kept all whitewear white, and it is important to remember that the more intricate the stitches on any piece of cloth, the more difficult it is to iron. Leisure time and servants not only permitted upper class women to produce prodigious amounts of exquisitely decorated wear for bed, body, table, and frequently just for show; they also guaranteed that these luxuries could be maintained.

Between the Great Tradition of a courtly aristocracy in Renaissance Italy and Sicily, and the rising commitment to embroidery among Villamaura peasants and artisans in the late nineteenth and early twentieth centuries, was a process of class formation, which, as elsewhere in Europe, elevated a landed bourgeoisie, or gentry, into a mediational position between local, rural populations, and metropolitan centers of power and prestige. A brief summary of this process for Sicily best begins with the early 1800s, when European, especially English, capital combined with policies of the Neapolitan Bourbons, then rulers of the island, to create a capitalist market in land. For the next several decades, families of diverse but often humble origin began to accumulate land; they formed the core of the so-called *ceto civile,* the "civilized people" who were Sicily's version of a gentry class.

At first the rise of the *ceto civile* contradicted the interests of a preexisting aristocracy, but the contradiction was more apparent than real, for bourgeois landholdings were rarely gained at aristocratic expense so much as they were carved from other sources: from state expropriations of ecclesiastical and communal domain on the one hand; from peasant indebtedness on the other. As displaced peasant rebels increasingly threatened the *civili* from below, this rising group assimilated to the class above them, not only politically and through marriage alliances, but by emulating an aristocratic life style. From at least the late 1860s, the main difference between the new gentry and the old aristocracy was in the scale of this style and where it was lived. For the *ceto civile* carried out its version of elite behavior in the confines of the rural and interior towns whereas earlier holders of large properties usually resided for most of the year in cities, at the courts of kings and princes, and abroad.

Happily for the ambitions of the *civili,* the nineteenth century was a time of substantial agrarian transformation which was Sicily's version of the second agricultural revolution. Again foreign capital and government policy played key roles, in this case converting land once used for extensive, trans-humant grazing into more intensively cultivated wheat fields and vineyards and, in south-central Sicily, into sulphur mines as well. Until the agricultural depression of the 1880s and 1890s, viable markets for grain, vineyards, and sulphur gave the rural bourgeoisie a generous financial base, if not for capitalizing their holdings, then at least for bringing civilization to the hinterland.

And this they did. The house cadaster of Villamaura shows that by the late 1870s, gentry families had already commissioned the construction of houses whose complex ground plans conformed to criteria recognized as *"civile"* throughout Italy and Europe. Articulated by Palladio, the great sixteenth-century architect of the Veneto, these criteria dictated that stables and storerooms should be totally separate from the residential quarters of the owners, even if in the same building, and that the architecture of the residential quarters should express the opposition of "nature" and "culture" wherever possible. Similar ideas were applied to the body, whose natural functions were camouflaged by fashionable clothes, chosen according to season, hour of the day, activity being pursued, and so on.[23] In dressing themselves, and their houses, no less than in the domain of architecture, the urbane *civili* insisted upon layers between layers, and here a proliferation of decencies was essential. Not only was the use of the handkerchief more hygienic than blowing one's nose in one's sleeve—to take a graphic example marvelously embroidered upon by Elias[24]—but, as Balsamo had urged, linens of all kinds "enhance and adorn the civilized life." From the *civile* point of view, the more decorated these linens were, the more this was true.

Civile families in late nineteenth-century Villamaura had occasional live-in servants plus dependent women who came to their houses on a more or less regular basis to sew, wash floors, and nurse infants. Other women took sewing or children into their own homes while laundresses *(lavandai)* washed the linens of the rich in local streams. By the 1870s and 1880s, there were bakeries and pasta "factories," which produced daily allotments of bread and noodles for those who could afford them, so one imagines that *civile* women had abundant leisure time to embroider.

Women of other classes were different in this regard for, although according to oral histories taking us back to the turn of the century, wives of rich peasants hired poor girls for heavy housework and running errands, plus seamstresses to come into their houses and sew, these wives, and the wives of other peasants and artisans, made their own bread and pasta, nursed their own children, and did their own laundry (unless they were sick). How was it that so many of them, following the example of the *civili,* also became devotees of the needle arts? Part of the answer to this question appears later on, in a discussion of women's work. For the moment we need to follow the class formation process to the point where non-*civile* groups also experienced a rise in their standard of living.

A well-known corollary of rural bourgeois ascendance is peasant proletarianization; this occurred quite markedly in Sicily after the expropriation of the church and common lands in the 1860s. Yet peasant impoverishment was not the only consequence of the growing *civile* monopoly of local power. The expansion of this class both numerically, and as status-conscious consumers, brought in its wake a series of effects that improved the life conditions for middle groups, too. Artisans, for example, grew more numerous and more skilled in large part because, given the lack of roads and railroads, most of the things with which the *civili* adorned themselves and their houses were crafted locally. Better-off peasants, too, benefitted from *civile* expansion, among other ways by providing luxury foods and tobacco for tables of the gentry class.

These groups and others just below them on the ladder of wealth and status were, however, extremely vulnerable to the agricultural depression that engulfed Europe in the 1870s when American wheat, cheaply produced by mechanical means and transported by steamships, crossed the Atlantic, and to the economic dislocations of the 1880s and 1890s, which resulted from the transatlantic flow of Louisiana sulphur and the complete collapse of the wine grape market, due to diseased vines and French competition. In the long run, therefore, out-migration was the basis for upward mobility among non-*civile* groups.

Contrary to a common assumption that migrants from southern Italy and Sicily were overwhelmingly landless day laborers is the recent discovery by historians that artisans and better-off peasants participated too.[25] After all, the multiplier effects of *civile* expansion worked rapidly in reverse once the grain, sulphur, and vineyard economy was undermined. Another revision of once common assumptions stems from mounting evidence that perhaps a third of all migrants to America returned to their homeland, some of them several times. Finally, although migrants' remittances are impossible to follow with precison, it is clear that they played a decisive role in the Sicilian economy after 1900—above all as a cash reserve for peasants and artisans.

Reserve cash facilitated the purchase of land, so that gradually the number of small holdings increased vis-à-vis the number of vast estates. Especially impressive were the changes in peasant and artisan patterns of consumption made possible by remittance money. Even before World War I, members of these "middle sectors" began to build or add on to houses, and to acquire more diversified wardrobes and household furnishings. Interviews with survivors and descendants of that era portray the change as another aspect of civilization coming to the hinterland. That rich and middle peasants and artisans adopted the practice of embroidering trousseau was in this sense merely an extension of the modeling behavior that engaged them as a general rule.

TEXTILE ARTS AND THE SECLUSION OF WOMEN

Even though a process of class formation and status emulation can tell us a great deal about the ever-wider distribution of embroidered decencies in Sicilian households after the mid-1800s, it does not fully explain why embroidery became central to trousseau. For one thing, history provides too many cases in which elite styles were reversed or rejected, ascetic movements nourished, counter cultures born, for emulation or modeling ever to be a sufficient cause of anything. Furthermore, to conclude that the downward circulation of embroidery and lacemaking was simply the consequence of upward mobility and "nouveau riche" excess is to overlook the labor requirements of needlework—requirements that once restricted such work to an elite domain. Posed as a problem of labor allocation, the ever-wider distribution of lace and embroidery in late nineteenth century Sicily becomes a corollary of the distribution of commercially manufactured cloth which in this period displaced an array of homespuns, and liberated nonelite mothers and daughters from the loom.

Let us return to the lists of peasant trousseaux which Salomone-Marino and Pitrè collected for the first few decades of the 1800s. By far the most numerous of the 35 to 40 items making up these lists were textiles and these ranged along a continuum from cloth intended for daily use to a special wedding dress. Purchased finery predominated in this dress: damasked silk from the famed Sicilian industries of the coastal cities, especially Messina, which was dyed with reliable dyestuffs (imported cochineal and indigo, or a domestic copper-sulphate derivative used with an alum mordant to produce a marvelous "peacock" blue-green). Portions of the costume, especially the bodice, were embellished with gold and silver thread, pieces of lace or macramé work in silk. Finally, a worked, sometimes inlaid, silver belt cinched it at the waist.[26]

In addition to the festival or wedding dress, purchased luxury fabrics such as silk or velvet (in one case Tibetan wool) figured in mantles and shawls, some of which were fringed, trimmed with gold thread or ribbon. Most of the other textiles—the necessities of daily use such as aprons, skirts, and whitewear for bed and table, were handloomed. Indeed, some trousseaux included lengths of cloth not as yet made up into particular articles.[27] Descriptions of this cloth, as well as of skirts, sheets, and so on mention the fibers of which they were made, the fineness of the weave, whether the weave was patterned in any way, and whether the cloth had been dipped in a home-prepared dye bath. From the evidence available, it appears that imported linen and cotton threads entered homewoven fabrics only to a very limited extent; domestic wool was also unusual except in shawls and for mattress stuffing. Domestic linen existed but was rare, due to problems of linen cultivation, and domestic cotton likewise. By far the most common cloths were of homegrown and homespun hemp, or hemp mixed with cotton to make fustians. When such cloth was woven without pattern or stripe, it was called *tela di casa ordinaria*—ordinary, homemade cloth.[28]

Not only did trousseaux of the early nineteenth century emphasize handloomed textiles; they included looms and spinning equipment as a general rule. For in those days, a good wife was a good weaver, so much so that it was customary for prospective mothers-in-law to find pretexts for discovering the weaving skills of their son's betrothed before the wedding date was fixed. A proverb said that if, on a surprise visit, the girl were found relaxing, she would be a lazy wife. If she were found eating, one could expect her to ruin the groom with her gluttony. But if she were found weaving, then she would be exemplary, like the wife who is quoted in Bennetti-Ventura's study of Sicilian textiles: "From the time I was 14 to 50, I dressed myself, my brothers, my children and the children of those with cloth made by my own hands."[29] Peasant women who were ill-prepared for such work were little sought-after; another old proverb likened them to the white crow (*corvo bianco*).[30]

The shift from homespun to machine-made cloth for clothing, tablewear, and bedding was both rapid and thorough. The following observation makes this point:

> Were all weddings made in such a way? Yes, all, because in those days there was not a family which did not have so many looms in motion, so many daughters who were inside, and the youngest wound the spools. No one would have married a girl who did not know how to weave, no one.
>
> Today, this custom has fallen almost entirely into disuse;

> because the industry of weaving is no longer in the hands of our peasant women; the cloth of foreigners has been formidably competitive, and the houses where weaving still takes place are few.[31]

Nevertheless, the displacement of domestic weaving did not occur everywhere or in all sectors at the same time. For one thing, women continued to wear homespuns for quite a while after men adopted the *stilo inglese*—English style tailored suits which became fashionable in Sicily in the late nineteenth century. Men of the gentry class owned such suits earlier and in greater number than did peasants, although better-off peasants in Villamaura had tailored pants, jackets, and vests at least as far back as 1890. Towns also changed differentially. Those situated at lower altitudes and in close proximity to the transportation network—rudimentary as this was until the 1900s—experienced the "formidable competition" of commercially produced cloth considerably in advance of towns that were remote. Villamaura, at 300 m above sea level and on the road connecting Corleone with Sciacca, fell into this category, whereas a more isolated neighboring community that I visited several times did not.

The contrast between these two settlements is interesting. In the remote mountain town, there are still a few working looms in the 1960s and although by then women wove only rustic saddle bags, they could explain how linen and hemp were cultivated, soaked, and beaten into malleable fibers, how it took 15-20 days of dawn-to-dusk weaving for the mothers and daughters, rotating at the loom, to produce the three lengths of cloth that made one sheet when sewn together—more days if the weave were fine. In Villamaura, by contrast, no one had firsthand experience with the cultivation of fibers, except briefly during World War II and, although many women had spun wool for coarse wartime sock-knitting, none with whom I spoke knew how to weave. Older informants, attempting to date when looms were last used, envisioned their grandmothers at them, and not their mothers. In fact, there appear to be no surviving looms in Villamaura. People there characterize residents of the neighboring mountain town as "*meno evoluto*," which means "less evolved" or backward. They say the best index of this is that the women there work outdoors rather than at the civilized indoor task of embroidery. Mountain women "*vanno in campagna*"—go out into the countryside—among other things to tend and process the locally produced fiber crops that Villamaura women gave up long ago.

These impressions, gathered during field work, of the differences between two communities, echo the conclusion of Cocchiara that ultimately weaving survived only in the mountainous zones of Messina and Trapani provinces in Sicily, Calabria, and Sardinia.[32] Elsewhere the expression "tela di casa" became an unflattering nickname (an *injuria)*. Vital statistics kept by municipal governments since 1820 in Sicily, include occupational information on men and women, and also permit tracing locally specific change. The data which I have for Villamaura reveal that a male weaver (a *telandaro)* who married in 1850 had become a cloth merchant by 1866 when his sixth child was born. Between then and 1881, four such merchants appeared in the sampled marriages (1850-1851, 1860-1861, 1870-1871, 1880-1881) alone. That these dealers were important is suggested by the fact that all married daughters of landed gentry or professionals, even though their fathers and mothers had been of artisan or (rich) peasant status. Since families generally attempted upward mobility through daughters, as for example in Lampedusa's famous novel The Leopard, these cases of an opposite pattern must have attracted a great deal of attention.

The Villamaura sample tells us that around 1866-1867, town clerks began recording the occupations of women married to peasants, shepherds, and artisans as "industrious" (*industriosa*); previously they had listed no occupations at all. In 1866, a woman who had married a stonecutter in 1850, appeared in the birth act of her fourth child as a seamstress (a *cucitrice*). This designation would be worth a detailed investigation. In the sample of families available to me now it reappeared in two birth acts in 1877 and then became general for the wives of virtually all artisans and better-off peasants (*agricoltori* or *burgisi*) in the mid-1880s—a decade when women in the neighboring mountain town were listed as *filatrici* or spinners. *Cucitrici* of the 1880s put seams in shirts and trousers. My informants thought that they did this as outworkers for local tailors, as well as for their own families, some perhaps with the aid of a sewing machine.[33]

The proliferation of *cucitrici* in Villamaura, beginning slowly in the late 1860s and expanding rapidly around 1883-1884, charts the penetration of commercial cloth. Significantly these dates correspond to important changes in policy at the level of the newly unified Italian state. For example, in the mid-1860s internal tariff barriers were dismantled to encourage a freer circulation of goods, including imports from abroad; in the 1880s, a national protective tariff nurtured the development of North Italian textile industries. Moreover, throughout these years, national policy directed both domestic and foreign capital into road and railroad construction—a transportation network being essential to the formation of a national market.[34] Villamaura had no accessible railhead until the twentieth century, but links by cart to Palermo and other coastal cities improved somewhat earlier. Cart drivers and retail merchants made up 1.1% of our 1850-51 marriage cohort. By 1870-1871 their number had risen to 4.5% and by 1880-1881 to 8%.

What with cloth merchants and carters, the operations of the market and the policies of the state, commercially produced textiles were finding their way into the Sicilian interior in even more lengths and widths after, say, 1870. Among these textiles was sheeting, for the most part machine-made cotton, some of it mixtures of cotton and other fibers.[35] As spinning and weaving declined, women applied highly elaborate needlework to this factory produced and commercially distributed cloth.[36]

In many respects, the transition is hardly remarkable. Embroidery had long existed in the upper class, as well as for the limited purpose of decorating the wedding dress. The skills that it requires are partially transferable from weaving; both necessitate an early acquaintance with the properties of different fibers and with sewing. According to women in Villamaura, learning to sew always precedes learning other textile arts. Yet the question remains why women, liberated from one kind of domestic chore should have taken up another one, especially one whose products were apparently less useful, and at a historical juncture when the Sicilian economy was losing its capacity to earn foreign exchange. If status emulation is not to bear the entire burden of explanation, what else was going on?

One might hypothesize that embroidery and lace-making evolved as a kind of make-work that ensured continuity in the division of labor by sex. Given its location and history, Sicily participated in the Mediterranean culture of honor and shame. As a set of structures and codes, this culture is familiar. Women brought status to their families in the degree that they were "pure": virgins at marriage, chaste as wives, continent as widows, and in general secluded from a public social life. If anything, hours spent at embroidery encouraged these virtues even more than spinning and weaving because when women worked on factory-made cloth, they no longer had anything to do with the cultivation and harvesting of fiber crops, tasks that had previously engaged them in cooperative endeavors with men outside the home.

I will argue that, like the status emulation hypothesis, the "make-work" hypothesis is not sufficient. Nevertheless, it has some real virtues which will be examined first in relation to married, or potentially married, women, then in relation to young girls before they marry. Regarding adult women, the disappearance of spinning and weaving added up to many hours of spare time, especially if one includes the hours of a growing number of women who could not marry because migration removed more males than females from the marriage market. By their very quantity, these hours were at least a theoretically serious threat to cultural continuity since they could have been allocated to work of the sort that men did, or to a search for pleasure outside the home. That these things did not happen on a significant scale may have a direct explanation: when the commodities which had been developed for export during the nineteenth century ceased to be viable, investors withdrew their capital and failed to encourage the production of anything else. Yet it is possible that this failure to consider alternatives was influenced by the perception that in Sicily, only the poorest women could be considered part of the labor pool. Other women were too committed to demonstrating their family's honor through the preparation of elaborate trousseau.

An interesting term to follow in the vital statistics records is *casalinga,* meaning housewife, a woman who lives at home without exercising another profession or occupation.[37] During the 1890s and early 1900s, some Villamaura wives of better-off peasants and artisans continued to appear in the marriage and birth registers as *cucitrici* but an increasing number were called *casalinghe.* Furthermore, whereas the wives of middle to poor peasants and shepherds had previously appeared as "industrious" or "peasant," many of them also acquired the label *casalinga* after 1890. In the 1910 and 1920 marriage cohorts, almost all women received this designation, except for women in the gentry class who, like their husbands, were called *civile,* and a few women of the peasant class who were extremely poor.

The *Grande Dizionario Battaglia* clarifies the normative message conveyed by the term "*casalinga*": a housewife who "loves to stay in the house, live in the bosom of her own family, occupying herself with domestic affairs, with the education of children, seeking refuge from rowdy entertainment." Literary citations assembled to illustrate this point include a few in which handwork or needlework symbolize a wife's resistance to the temptations of frivolity and vice. In the *Enciclopedia Italiana,* the term is equated with *casalina,* which means either a homewoven garment of unrefined cotton with a blue or black background or bottom, or a linen weaving frame.[38] "*Inga,*" however, is a suffix meaning "of the"—in this case of the house. If *casalinga* conveys a central idea, it is that being "of the house" is equivalent to having a serious occupation or profession, perhaps partly because of domestic textile production.

Turning now to nubile women, the link between textiles and restrained sexuality is even more explicit, as the English word "spinster" reminds us. This is because Christianity (other great religions, too) often equates industrious dedication to spinning, weaving, and embroidery with virginity. Already in the Middle Ages, cloistered nuns wove and decorated clerical vestments and altar cloths. As repositories of skill and design, convents ever since have taught girls both clothwork and morals even in such out-of-the-way places as Villamaura. There, before the suppression of religious orders in 1866, a Collegio of Santa Maria instructed "respectable girls" how to embroider in silk and gold as well as pursue "domestic and manual labor, both necessary and ornamental, which a good mother of a family needed to know."[39] In 1873, the state permitted the sisters of this Collegio to continue to train girls under the guise of an *opera pia* or charity; this training came to focus increasingly on embroidery.

According to Christian teaching, the production of beautiful and refined cloth is an act of religious devotion, no less than are vows of chastity. The two often go together as we see in the lives of "house nuns"—devout women who, although they belong to no official religious community, never marry and spend their days embroidering for home and church. Other examples abound in the biographies of female saints such as Saint Agatha, the Christianized Penelope, whose following is considerable among Sicilian women. She continually put off her suitor, much to her father's dismay, on the grounds that she could not marry him until she had finished weaving a certain cloth. Agatha wove by night and day but "her woman's work was never done," and instead of getting married she became the patron saint of spinners and weavers.[40]

In the legend of Saint Agatha, devotion to weaving meant the postponement of marriage, but in the lives of women in Sicily, embroidery correlated with delayed marriage more closely than did weaving. This is because the expansion of embroidery at the end of the nineteenth century roughly coincided with the demographic transition from large to small families, a transition that depended in part on marriage age. According to our family-reconstitution study for Villamaura, women's age at marriage was relatively low in all classes until the 1890s. After that, it was low among the poorest peasants who married in their late teens, but averaged 25 years or more in other groups.

In the early decades of the nineteenth century, women entered marriage with spinning and weaving equipment, tested skills as weavers, and some cloth. It was expected that they would produce many more lengths of the same as wives and mothers. In contrast, the embroidery regime of the end of the century, which was associated with a later age at marriage, made a distinction between work done before and after the marriage. Before, a young girl embroidered her entire trousseau, being careful to project an image of herself as both industrious and modest; after marriage she did little if any embroidery, except for the layettes and baptismal dresses of newborn children and, when time permitted, occasional pieces for gifts.[41] After marriage, women's primary task was to manage their daughters' trousseaux. Thus embroidery was above all an activity and symbol of virgin girlhood, the more so as it was usually white on white.[42]

TROUSSEAU AS TREASURE

Like our review of class formation and status emulation, this picture of women's work as an aspect of women's "value" illuminates the embroidery problem. It also complements, without detracting from, an explanation for this practice based on rivalry for status. Indeed, ethnographic data indicate that, in the status hierarchy for women, types of work and degrees of purity went hand in hand. Thus in Chapman's account, young girls "with status pretensions" substituted embroidery for knitting and weaving and assumed they would "never bake their own bread or do their own laundry." At the same time, status-conscious peasant and artisan women remained "in complete isolation" where they embroidered or supervised embroidery, and wore "veils to Church in imitation of (the) wealthy."

In all of these groups, women married late, sometimes later than 30.[43]

Interviews with elderly women from very poor families in Villamaura brought out a different complex of traits associated with the lower end of a female hierarchy: For these women, the most time-consuming activity was to save their children from starvation and this necessitated all kinds of low status work. They made brooms and cording for itinerant merchants and local mediators who put out the raw materials—the processed leaves and stalks of local plants. They gathered wild vegetables on what remained of public lands, followed the men on the fields at harvest time in order to pick up stray stalks of grain, and ground this grain on their own stones to avoid an onerous tax on machine-milled flour. The time employed in home-milling was to some extent compensated by time gained from cooking and baking, because the stone ground flour was too course for pasta or bread and tended to be eaten as a porridge, called *pitirru*.

Girls from very poor families often worked as maids to earn money for dowry and their mothers worked as laundresses to enhance the same fund. But sons' earnings went to the mother for food rather than sheeting; thus most families could manage at best a minimum trousseau for their daughters. Few hoped for upward mobility through female offspring; on the contrary, the sooner a daughter married and joined an independent household, the better. Sometimes—poignantly illustrating Pitrè's observation that "marriages of the poor create new poor"—a mother was able to give the last of her own infants to a married daughter to nurse, that daughter having already begun to have children.[44]

Early marriage and the pressure of poverty stood in the way of learning to sew—let alone embroider—and many women recall with bitterness that for them, clothes were made by piecing together the hand-me-downs of others whereas handwork consisted only in making brooms. In their view, having done no embroidery was worse than a social stigma; it confirmed the *civile* ideology that day laborers lived like animals, crowded into one or two rooms with their donkey and, as Malthus thought, breeding without control. Clearly, proletarian women had no honor, whereas women who embroidered did, and their embroidered trousseaux symbolized not only this crucial fact, but the layers between them and proletarianization.

By considering the cultural connection between certain kinds of handwork and sexual restraint, we have deepened our perspective on social status. The owner of embroidery and lace emitted more than a claim to participation in the Great Traditions of a civilization; there was also a message of assurance that her family would not sink, as it were, beyond the pale. One detects the familiar concerns of a "petty bourgeoisie": (*a*) how to distance themselves from those who, in an earlier generation, were their class equals; (*b*) how to cope with the unsettling reality that, were it not for a few lucky breaks, they could be proletarians, too; (*c*) how to find in their preoccupation with honor a justification for screening out the domestic tragedies associated with a neighbor's impoverishment.

But why, after all of this, was embroidery a central symbol of social position? Why not establish the same point with the wide range of consumer goods that factory production and improved transportation made ever more readily, and cheaply, available in the twentieth century? These goods conferred status, too. I raise this question because I am dissatisfied with the conclusion that embroidery was make-work, however much it distinguished the embroiderer. This seems to me to distort both women's commitment to it, and the central role that it played in marriage exchange.

As we have seen, bride and groom contributed different things to their new household. Against her status goods he brought productive resources—if not land, then at least the strength, social relations, and agricultural implements with which to earn a livelihood from the land or, if he were an artisan, the tools and skills of a trade. Yet there is no indication that her contribution, while different, was inferior to his. In writing about the Sarakatsani, Campbell suggests that the addition of sheep or gold sovereigns to a traditional dowry of household goods has improved women's chances to marry up, but this trend appeared only after 1945.[45] Pitkin's study and other accounts of Italy are quite explicit that in the past, *corredo* alone could attract a spouse of equal or superior status.[46] Moreover, even though trousseau predominates over other goods in many Mediterranean dowry systems, ethnographers frequently comment that in the household, wife and husband enjoy matched status and use reciprocal terms of address.[47] In a Sicilian proverb, "The man is the soul of the house. A good wife is the primary wealth of the house."[48]

One kind of evidence that embroidered "beds" constituted a store of wealth lies in the ritual of the *stima.* The professional who examined assembled trousseau before a wedding used well established criteria to estimate value. Regarding the raw materials, linen outranked cotton, which outranked hemp; moreover, Belgian linen was superior to Irish linen, which was in turn superior to Italian. Silk thread had more value than cotton thread in embroidery. The *stimatrice* also examined workmanship, judging both the difficulty of the stitches and the precision of their execution. But most important, she looked at overall design, because different design sequences carried different values. These sequences were the heritage of Renaissance Italy and Sicily, also of eighteenth century France; they were kept and transmitted by cloistered nuns who, in Villamaura, sold them for a fee.

Designs were also available from local women who had received training as *disegnatrici* in Palermo, and from specialized journals and pattern booklets. Publications of this type have long contributed to the standardization of embroidery and lace-making in Europe, their existence dating back to the second quarter of the sixteenth century when wood-engraved printing came into its own. As a rule, pattern booklets instruct women not in creating or transferring designs, so much as in rigorously copying them by counting threads in the cloth or mesh ground (a process called embroidery *a fili contati* or *à points comptés).* Some of the designs to be copied were produced by men, but women authored many of the best known sequences. Such sequences usually originated in key centers of textile manufacture such as Flanders and Venice in the sixteenth century; Milan since the late 1800s. These centers gave place names to particular patterns or stitches which the booklets then carried even to peasant households in far-away villages.[49]

Some designs emphasized cut-work, done with sharp scissors but without an embroidery hoop, and relatively easy to execute. (Minimum "beds," if they were embroidered at all, were usually ornamented with cut-work.) More complicated and time consuming was drawn work (*sfilato*), transitional between embroidery and lace in that it involved removing threads from a woven ground. A Sicilian version of *sfilato* gained a continental reputation in the fourteenth century and is highly prized in *corredo* to this day.[50] Other *sfilato* patterns also had Renaissance roots, but in Northern Italy, not Sicily. Among the most prestigious and valued designs were those which incorporated the Venetian rose-point; open mesh cloth embroidered with palm, rose, peacock, or geometric motifs; and appliqués of Tuscan pillow lace. Significantly, there was little individual experimentation or artistic expression in trousseau preparation; most girls, guided by their mothers, adhered closely to the established designs.[51]

The standardized criteria used by a *stimatrice* to estimate the value of trousseau in lire or onze obviously had some relation to a sphere of exchange, and the fact that designs with continental reputations weighed heavily in her calculus suggests that this sphere transcended not only a local arena, but ultimately, Sicily as well. One can question how much exchange value items of trousseau actually had—according to John Davis, not very much. "*Corredo,*" he writes, "is a poor sort of investment; it does not carry interest, nor does it have great liquidity; it is hard to sell it, and impossible to secure a loan with."[52]

Davis, however, is reporting a contemporary situation, and perhaps he has, as a reference, modern forms of saving against a rainy day: bank accounts, stocks and bonds, insurance policies, union benefits, and presumably fool-proof government programs covering crop damage, retirement, war injuries, earthquakes, and so on. In the period of concern to us here, these forms of long-run security were rudimentary at best; many of them have come into being for the Italian South and Sicily only with the considerable expansion of state institutions after World War II. Moreover, the period in question closely followed the breakup of a number of religious orders, which in earlier centuries had supplemented family strategies for "ultimate" survival.

What existed instead was a pyramid of patron-client relations whose ability to deliver protection and welfare depended heavily on personal criteria, and on the financial solvency of the *civile* class. Big spenders and poor investors, this class was shaken in times of trouble, too. In other words, in the late nineteenth and early twentieth centuries, most families were on their own to meet the crises of life—the loss of a work animal, an expensive litigation against encroachments on property, the untimely death of a breadwinner. Such were the events that raised their debt level and led them to the brink of the abyss where survival meant selling off productive resources and finding a daily, or hourly, wage. That people who reached this point often joined the migration stream is less significant than that they joined it as lumpen proletarians with no "monetary refuge" to ease the transition. Families that had such a refuge in some ways resembled states, which is perhaps why in wedding ceremonies bride and groom were the symbolic equivalents of a king and queen; their attendants the equivalent of a court.

In Villamaura, I was told that embroidered sheets and bed covers, especially the most valued and least used, saved a number of families from disaster. The point is not that "beds" were regularly exchanged; on the contrary, selling or pawning them was the last resort—a desperate, almost immoral, economic necessity. Yet oral histories reveal that sometimes women pawned whitewear at local grocery or yardgood stores to purchase food or sheeting for a daughter's trousseau. Itinerant merchants secretly negotiated with women who were eager for a "family allowance" but ashamed that anyone should know they would trade *corredo* to get it. Church sponsored pawn shops, the *Monte di Pietà,* dating back to the seventeenth century, made loans against whitewear, too. I also heard stories of creditors bursting in on troubled families and opening their linen chests, the contents of which had no legal protection against the claims of third parties—unlike other components of dowry that creditors could not touch.[53]

Most of the stories concerned families that had few resources to begin with; there were exceptions, however, reminiscent of those which a Philadelphia pawn broker reported in an interview with the *Literary Digest* in 1921. According to his account, "a reputable pawn broker can be described as a poor man's banker," but the rich who borrow from banks nevertheless sometimes ring the bell at night, carrying the family silver and other "ancient heirlooms" under their arms. Their purpose is to raise money to pay back debts which unlucky ventures have caused to become outstanding.[54] One should not imagine, in other words, that better-off families were immune to crises. Their vulnerability to disease was nearly as great as anyone's until the 1700s, and after 1789, revolutions could do them in. Various accounts of upper-class dowries from earlier centuries suggest that as a rule of thumb, new households were formed with *corredo* that was commensurate with the value of immovable property, or a family was not worthy of its name.[55] Perhaps we should think of trousseau as a store of value that protected not only family members, but also family assets, providing the flexibility to meet crises by pawning or selling wealth instead of land.

The negotiability of whitewear ultimately depended on whether claimants, creditors, and pawnbrokers could resell their catch. Probable buyers in the stories told by Villamaura women were mothers engaged in trousseau preparation in distant communities, some in continental Italy. The size of trousseaux among the *civili* must have helped enlarge the sphere of exchange since no girl, however late she married, could embroider 50 or more beds by herself. A close study of the connections between landed families, the cloistered convents where nuns embroidered in part for wealthy clients, and the religious pawn shops, might further validate the hypothesis that, although *biancheria* was largely produced for use within the home, it was also potentially exchangeable for cash or food.[56]

To the extent that whitewear was a potentially liquid resource, it served as more than a symbolic layer between a peasant or an artisan family and proletarianization. It could constitute a real economic buffer when crises threatened, much like the wealth objects suitable for "emergency conversion" in Africa.[57] In this context, the distinction between embroidered goods and consumer goods becomes clear, for although the latter also confer status, their time to depreciation is practically zero. It is important, in other words, to differentiate among *types* of prestige goods, or status symbols. Consumer goods may attract more attention and admiration than old lace because they are more fashionable, but it is among other things their fashion-bound quality that contributes to their rapid obsolescence. In contrast, old lace, especially if it conforms to well established patterns, keeps its value even as it appears out of date, and can be traded for "survival" in troubled times.

Lace, embroidery, and needlepoint fall into the range of prestige goods best characterized as wealth objects, or valuables. Significantly, in Sicily, the ideological complex that conflated virginity and delayed marriage with handwork of this sort, also cautioned women against "frivolity and vice." Many fashionable clothes and furnishings entered the marriage exchange system as gifts, which the spouses gave each other, or received from friends and relatives, but these goods were like the purchased cosmetics and perfumes which Salomone-Marino complained, already in 1879, were corrupting the "virginal fragrance" of the bride.[58] They lacked the ageless value of precious things.[59]

But precious things are varied too, and a final step in this attempt to discover "why embroidery" is to contrast valuables among themselves. Recall that in the trousseau lists of the early nineteenth century there were a number of wealth objects—in particular silk, gold, and silver—associated with the wedding dress. Other items, not referred to as yet, included gold rings and earrings, a silver hair brush, and a rosary inlaid with pearl. The daughter of a carter from a Palermo suburb brought into her marriage several copper pots, plus a bronze mortar, while better-off peasant girls had amber and coral.[60] Objects such as these did not disappear from trousseaux toward the end of the century, but it seems to me that their presence was less noticeable as time went on. The wedding belt, for example, gave way to a comparable, but much smaller, symbol—the wedding ring. Already in Palermo of the late nineteenth century, a white wedding dress worn with garlands of orange blossoms replaced the polychrome and damasked silk costume ornamented with gold buttons and gold thread.[61] (In the interior towns, however, this transition took longer).[62] The "traditional" costume of silk and gold depreciated much less rapidly than the "modern" one of machine made cloth and flowers, even though the latter became more fashionable and prestigious.

It appears that little is known of the processes by which peasants and artisans (as distinct from noblemen and gentry) came to own significant preciosities—especially articles of gold and silver, and the finely woven silks of urban craftshops.[63] We usually assume that sumptuary laws prevented the diffusion of these things. Nor do we have good accounts of how such goods were removed from modest households. Regarding nineteenth-century Sicily, one wonders how nongentry families experienced a tax burden that not only increased steadily with Italian Unification, but was among the most regressive in Europe;[64] how a severe shortage of coin, coupled with a rising pace of circulation, affected them, particularly when the government issued decrees urging private citizens and ecclesiastical bodies to cash in plate for money and other concessions;[65] how they managed when the creation of a national debt out of several regional debts in the 1860s severely disrupted public finance, or when the depression of the last quarter of the nineteenth century triggered bankruptcies in agriculture and industry. These were events that would deplete the family coffers.

Regarding silk, Mack Smith has noted that rich Sicilians preferred French imports while poorer people "ceased to be able to afford it as their standard of living went down." This loss of a home market in turn weakened the Sicilian silk industry, despite the introduction of Jacquard looms in midcentury and, with the elimination of internal tariffs in the 1860s, manufacturing totally collapsed, making silk even less accessible to peasants and artisans.[66]

Although information pertaining to precious metals and silks in peasant households is lacking, I draw attention to them because they differ from embroidery in a fundamental way. As a group they required virtually no labor on the part of the family possessing them—ornamentation of the wedding dress being a partial exception (unless lace and macramé trim were also purchased, which they may have been). And while these objects did contain "embodied" labor (labor expended at an earlier time) they also derived value from certain properties intrinsic to their "nature"—their rareness, beauty, luster, durability, and so on. In the history of textiles, there is support for the idea that these different components of value—natural beauty and rarity on the one hand, a considerable investment of labor on the other—interacted in patterned ways.

For example, there are numerous cases where intensification of cloth production occurred to meet a crisis of gold or silver drain. Governments, such as the familiar regimes of mercantilist Europe, often took pains to mobilize labor for textile manufacture because labor-intensive cloth exports could earn bullion abroad. Also intriguing is the repeated tendency of precious cloths to take the place of metals as a medium of exchange and store of value—that is, to assume money functions. Thus, precisely when bullion was scarce, the imperial court of China periodically declared silk and brocade (also porcelain and lacquer wear) to be "money."[67]

For a divergent, and yet similar, case, we can turn to Gambia (and other African countries) in the nineteenth century. There the Wolof wove cloth for exchange purposes when European contact made cowrie shells untenable by deflating their value, at the same time failing to introduce enough metal coins to fill the gap. According to Ames, the most beautiful of their cloths, pieces that were indigo-dyed with designs, did not circulate; their function was closer to treasure than to money.[68] Here a parallel can be found in the unique silks hoarded by the Chinese court, and in other famous textiles that filled the coffers of states, temples, monasteries, and churches everywhere. "The lily cannot hide in the garden," says a document of the Christian church called "Annals of the Virgin Saints,"

> for it is the flower of virgins (and) must deck the high altars. So with gold and silver and gems of the mine, they blaze in the chalice and . . . are curiously wrought in the mitre and the clasped cope, they glitter on the pastoral staff and processional cross; so with the work of the needle, the hanging, the frontal, the corporal, and the veil, all exercise the patient skill of the artist, all occupy the quiet hours of the convent.[69]

Yet different types of cloth approximated gold and silver in different ways. Closest were the textiles that were woven with gold and silver thread (actually very fine wire) and silk to form rich damasks and brocades. In these fabrics—early specialties of Oriental civilizations as far west as Byzantium—exotic fibers, metals, and dye-stuffs were a major component of value; so also were the rare skills of the drawloom weaver, usually an urban (male) specialist whose lengthy apprenticeship taught him how to manipulate colors and textures as he wove complicated designs. Even in ancient and medieval history, embroidered cloth was different, the critical factor in its production being tedious, patient work—neither terribly skilled nor requiring rich materials. In the words of Pauline Johnston, "countries such as Byzantium, Persia and Japan which at various times have attained a very high degree of skill in the production of decorated textiles, have always regarded embroideries very much in the light of a poor relation."[70]

Although embroidery and its close cousin, lace work, are potentially exquisite and highly reputed as fine arts, they developed as second bests to drawloom brocades that they were, at first, intended to imitate. Court-sponsored and urban embroidery industries (as distinct from household manufacture) came to perfection, in fact, in regions that were peripheral to the great civilizations, and also in those civilizations at the moment of their decline. Good examples of the former are England in the Middle Ages, and the Balkan peoples under Byzantine hegemony in the fourteenth and fifteenth centuries—especially the Balkan courts in Moldavia and Wallachia. In these regions, the conditions did not exist for silkworm cultivation and silk manufacture, but embroidery made it possible to elaborate indigenous cloths so that they looked like exquisite brocades. Indeed, "the ground material was often commonplace and embroidery covered it completely."[71] One is reminded of medieval convents in north Germany where white on white embroidery became "typical" because "of poverty, of lack of means. . .for the purchase of costly silk."[72] Peasant household production was similar, too. According to A. J. B. Wace, "in peasant art, embroidery is often employed as a home craft substitute for the luxurious woven silks of the rich and upper classes, and especially used to decorate the draperies demanded by social custom for trousseaux and festivals."[73]

With regard to declining civilizational centers, Johnston's study of Byzantine embroidery places great emphasis on *timing.* Almost unknown at the height of imperial development in the ninth and tenth centuries, when silk and brocade manufacture provided the foundation for an immense accumulation of bullion and slaves, embroidery industries developed in the wake of the Fourth Crusade.[74] At that juncture, the Venetians and Genoese extorted unfavorable trading agreements with Byzantium, which triggered the Empire's contraction. Imitative of drawloom weaving, embroiderers applied gold thread to lesser cloths through a method known as "laying and couching" and with time even the thread they used deteriorated in quality—becoming first gilded silver and then colored silk. Coincidentally, embroidery took on more intricate designs.[75] In other words, the balance sheet of exotic materials and rare skilled labor, as against hours of tedious needle pushing, shifted a notch toward the latter, much as happened when orientalized togas of rich stuffs gave way to embroidered robes with the decline of Rome after Diocletian.[76]

The origin of lace provides a special example of intensive labor becoming a source of value in lieu of precious materials at a point where those materials became less accessible. Developing out of embroidery, lace differs from it in a fundamental way. One embroiders on a piece of cloth, although the mesh of the weave can be opened considerably by drawing threads. Lace, on the other hand, requires the construction of its own ground or scaffolding by techniques that resemble knitting, knotting, and weaving. In other words, lace is created from air. And where European embroidery traditions, initially imported from Asia, often relied on threads of precious metal or colored silk, dyed with exotic dyestuffs, the inspiration for lace came from white thread embroidery on a white linen ground. Its attraction consisting in a play on open spaces instead of color, it required a bare minimum of valued materials. Significantly, its development in the sixteenth century was accomplished by women in domestic settings rather than men in urban workshops, while the first centers to produce lace in abundance were Northern Italy and Flanders—regions that had enjoyed a precocious economic growth during the Middle Ages but that were then losing ground to the hub of the emerging capitalist system in England and Holland.[77]

Embroidered cloth was a second cousin to hand-loomed brocade as a wealth object (just as brocade, although it approximated precious metals, was a second cousin to gold); this is reflected in the behavior of appropriators and pillagers when confronted with a choice. In the eyes of a nineteenth century needleworker for the Catholic Church in England, Henry VIII will go down in history as the world's greatest enemy of embroidery. His agents, in their zeal to transfer monastic property to king and gentry, ripped the gold thread off vestments and melted it down for coin![78] Greedier for the material than for the workmanship with which it was applied to the cloth, their preference has been echoed many times since, such as during Year Three of the French Revolution when 40 or 50 needlewomen at Angers were put to work picking gold and silver thread out of bed valances and canopies to be "sent to the smelting pots for the benefit of the nation. . ."[79]

A recent demonstration of the preference for valued materials over labor can be found in twentieth century Sicily. According to my sources in Villamaura, when a family was wealthy enough to purchase Belgian linen for dowry, the daughter did not embroider it because it was precious enough by itself. This suggests to me that if ordinary Sicilian families had been able to hang on to gold and silk in the course of the nineteenth century, they would have felt less compelled to commit so much of their women's time to embroidery.

CONCLUSIONS

In attempting to understand the centrality of embroidered "beds" in Sicilian marriage exchanges, the first step isolated this practice in time, for in fact it is not an old tradition except in the upper class. Class differences with regard to embroidery then led to a consideration of social mobility and status emulation as fundamental processes in the diffusion of the needle arts. A brief review of Sicilian social history in the nineteenth century showed that this was indeed a period when large-scale changes in land use and tenure produced new wealth, new occupational groups, new levels of consumer and status behavior on the local level.

The nineteenth century generated another source of change in the form of machine-made, factory-produced cotton and fustian textiles. As these yardgoods penetrated the peripheries of Europe and the world, they unhinged local and regional relations of production. One must not assume that their impact was everywhere the same, however. Sicily, and perhaps the Mediterranean generally, was a place where, prior to industrial textiles, the standards of cloth consumption were relatively high, and even among peasants included a range of decencies as well as basic clothes. Domestically produced cloth met these standards, as women allocated time to the cultivation and refinement of fiber crops, spinning, weaving, and even dyeing. The exception was silk, which was largely the product of specialized urban manufacture in Sicily, and which provided the fabric for festive wear. Machine-made textiles not only undermined the Sicilian silk industry; they also displaced the industries of the home.

The precipitous decline of home spinning and weaving liberated the hours that made it possible for peasants and artisans to emulate elites; what had earlier maintained the needle arts as an upper class monopoly was leisure time gained from slaves and servants. However, so many liberated hours could not in themselves account for the transition to embroidery, because too many other conditions were also changing. The Europe-wide depression of the late nineteenth century brought about a crisis of development: How could the various regions of England and the continent continue to compete in foreign markets, or even in their own, once the vast American cornucopia, fertilized by European capital, began to spill its surplus overseas? In Sicily this crisis underlay a spreading revolt among artisans and peasants, followed by heavy out-migration. One wants to know why, in the midst of dislocations of such severity, women stayed at home embroidering. The question becomes even more difficult when it is recognized that the demographic transition, an aspect of the crisis, considerably reduced the average number of childbearing years, particularly among those groups most committed to trousseau preparation.

An initial answer to the question focused on the cultural complex of honor and shame. According to this line of reasoning, embroidery, although beautiful and a source of prestige, was also make-work, as good as, or better than weaving for keeping nubile girls and the women who supervised them, out of trouble. Ethnographic observation confirms a symbolic association between embroidery and sexual restraint. That its principal "function" and hence "cause" was to underwrite female purity in a tumultuous age of change is another matter, however. For this conclusion overlooks the considerable and fascinating evidence that, far from being make-work, "beds" were a form of stored wealth that families could fall back on in emergencies. Girls who produced them took great care to duplicate standardized design sequences, and to prepare several pieces that, although they might be displayed, were destined for linen chests and not for use.

We have noted that, until quite late in the twentieth century, the long-run viability of Sicilian families and their defense against proletarianization necessitated possession of mobile wealth as well as productive resources, so much so that the marriage exchange system gave equal weight to both. Moreover, gold, silver, and precious silk became less accessible to peasants and artisans in the course of the 1800s, while modern forms of insurance and security would not become a reality in Sicily until the 1950s and 1960s. Dedication to embroidery was, in the long sweep of things, an "interim arrangement." Not only did it evolve naturally out of the earlier domestic role of women, and descend with equal ease from the consumption styles of the rich, but its development also conformed to a pattern for which history has many parallels: the pattern of creating value through intensification of labor, when control over rare and desired things declines. If the wealth thus created (from whole cloth, as it were), was inferior to more liquid forms such as gold, this is somewhat beside the point. For how many choices were there within the means of Sicilian peasants and artisans in the late nineteenth century?

To focus on trousseau as treasure is not to abandon the understanding that embroidery was an important status symbol, nor does such an emphasis contradict its association with chastity and purity. It does, however, suggest that symbols which are also material goods may be multifunctional. Historically, the industrial revolution and the capitalist world system that so rapidly advanced and diffused it, drove a wedge between status goods and valuables—a wedge that was previously unrealized. For in the past, most of the "things" that people, regardless of class position, were pleased to own and display were also potentially convertible, whereas today it is a proportionally ever smaller elite that enjoys the security of ornamenting its domestic surroundings with negotiable treasures (actual houses being at best a partial exception). Yet social scientists, themselves products of an industrial age, attribute to past status goods the same one-dimensional quality that characterizes such goods today—the quality of communicating and celebrating social position. And this, I think, leads to other oversimplifications: exaggerating the distinctions between goods produced for use and goods produced for exchange, and between prestige goods and necessities. Much of today's vocabulary in the social sciences in fact represents these categories not only as mutually exclusive, but as opposites, just as it encourages us to oppose domestic and public spheres of economic activity as women's and mens' work, respectively.

If we can generalize from this case study, until very recently items of trousseau were produced simultaneously for use and potential exchange; their content was at once ornamental and, when stored for emergency conversion, essential. The women who made and owned them, although they usually had little or no land, nevertheless contributed a critical resource to household viability; households as manufactories of cloth, which had exchange potential, were not wholly private domains. In each case, dichotomous categories are blurred and new kinds of relationship made apparent. We begin to see, for example, that the process of status emulation or filtering down of elite behavior was not just a matter of slavish imitation; it was at the same time a way for ordinary people to acquire goods that, should they ever have to be exchanged, would find ready takers because of their resemblance to elite goods whose spheres of exchange were worldwide.

In addition, we see that a cultural emphasis on sex segregation and female seclusion served both the symbolic end of demonstrating women's purity and the practical end of tying their labor down to looms and needles from which came treasures as well as decencies and clothes. Such observations prompt a reconsideration of persistent problems—for example, identifying the conditions that brought about the confinement of women to a domestic arena, and establishing the significance of dowry even when it contained no land.

They also influence the way we look at the present. In Sicily today, less cloth is embroidered and stored against a rainy day. Nor has *biancheria* retained its efficacy as a symbol of status, a prestigious gift, an object for display, having steadily lost ground to mass-produced consumer goods such as digital watches and ceramic wall tiles. Indeed, consumer goods now dominate wedding gifts and trousseaux. At first one wonders what role embroidery machines for home and factory have played in this transition. Early machines of this type appeared in Alsace before the end of the nineteenth century, but Lefébure, writing in the 1880s, argued that their impact on artistic handicrafts would only be temporary because "well-cared for handworks have. . .always been, and presumably always will be, wanted."[80]

Today a few women in Villamaura produce embroideries for sale on home machines but I do not think hand-embroidering has declined because of this competition. Its decline seems related to a substantial reallocation of women's time away from the needle arts and towards education and wage-earning occupations. Local markets for machine embroideries have grown as a result, and one begins to see a new interest in the kinds of craft that fill American magazines for homemakers: "Use Embroidery's Laziest Stitch to Style Up Your Table Settings," "Big, Bold Stitches," and so on.

In 1951, half as many girls as boys attended middle school in Villamaura, while only 48 of the 125 students completing secondary school were girls. In 1971, girls accounted for 46% of the *scuola media* diplomas, 49% of high school diplomas; there were also 15 young women with college degrees. Although education is no more a guarantee of employability in Sicily than it is in the United States, it has clearly taken the place of embroidered trousseau: In the eyes of most parents, it makes their daughters more marriageable than a hundred beds. It also makes women's contribution to the establishment of new households less different from men's than was true in the past—which is symptomatic of an overall erosion of a once thoroughgoing division of labor by sex. Thus, although some women still embroider, they do so as outworkers for merchants who introduce their handwork into a world market for tourist and "ethnic" wares.[81] Many other women have entered into commerce as small shopkeepers, or into bureaucracies as secretaries, and a growing number work beside men in agriculture. Their income, small as it is in relation to men's, helps underwrite the purchase of consumer goods.

What seems remarkable about all these changes is that they have occurred without much ado, and in a period of relative calm. Yet they constitute a reorientation of established cultural patterns that is far more dramatic than the shift from weaving to embroidery, which occurred in the context of capitalist penetration, severe depression, failed revolution, and mass migration at the end of the nineteenth century. Clearly there are lessons here about folk culture. It would seem that, even though economic and demographic pressures shake little traditions loose from their moorings and bring about alterations in their content, people do not necessarily abandon them unless or until the externally supported institutional matrix undergoes considerable expansion. In this particular case, at least, a wide range of suprafamilial institutions—for the most part creatures of the postwar state—now gives Sicilians the security they need to relax their dedication to cultural codes previously associated with the accumulation of treasure in family treasure chests.

This is not to imply, however, that public institutions work better to cushion crises than items of trousseau. Obviously more efficient, and less humiliating as a last resort, they are also much farther from home. So today, in Sicily, we find adult women, wives, and mothers, coping with application forms, sitting in offices, and demonstrating in the streets. Ironically, the time available for these means of pressing a faceless bureaucracy to respond to personal need is time gained from supervising their daughters' handwork and keeping up embroideries of their own.

REFERENCES

My analysis of trousseau grows out of a larger project that is concerned with class formation and demographic change in late nineteenth-century Sicily. Peter Schneider has been both a partner in this project and a key source of substantive and editorial criticisms of this chapter. I also received excellent criticisms and suggestions from Donna Gabaccia, Ashraf Ghani, and Patricia Torres; editorial assistance and encouragement from T.O. Beidelman, Joyce Riegelhaupt and Eric Wolf pointed out ways that I might tighten my argument, while Pamela Quagiotto and Pamela Wright helped me with linguistic evidence. Anthropology students at Yale University raised helpful questions after hearing my first draft in their Colloquium series. In addition to thanking these friends and colleagues, I wish to express my appreciation for many hours of conversation with Shirley Lindenbaum. Often touching on dowry systems as a problem for cross-cultural comparison our talks were the inspiration for worrying about trousseau.

1. J. Davis, *People of the Mediterranean: An Essay in Comparative Social Anthropology* (London, 1977), 43-54.

2. P. Schneider and J. Schneider, *Culture and Political Economy in Western Sicily* (New York, 1976).

3. D.S. Pitkin, ''Marital Property Considerations Among Peasants,'' *Anthropological Quarterly,''* 33(1960): 33-39.

4. J. Davis, *Land and Family in Pisticci* (London, 1973).

5. S. Silverman, *Three Bells of Civilization: the Life of an Italian Hill Town* (New York, 1975), 198.

6. M. Gömül, *Turkish Embroideries, XVI-XIX Centuries* (Istanbul, n.d.).

7. Quoted in G.C. Chapman, *Milocca: A Sicilian Village* (Cambridge, 1971), 30.

8. A recent doctoral dissertation on the cultural history of Sicilian migrants to America explores the implications of this method of registering ''houses'' for taxation, and includes data from the 1877 cadaster in Villamaura (see D. Gabaccia, ''Houses and People: Sicilians in Sicily and New York.'' Unpublished dissertation, University of Michigan, 1979).

9. As William Foote Whyte, summarizing the work of Pitrè, explained in some detail, the term ''peasant'' in Sicily referred to a range of occupations, minutely graded by status. In this context, it probably means better off, or middle, peasant, bordering on rich peasant or *burgise.* As a rule, the rich peasant either owned enough land to necessitate hiring day-laborers or sharecroppers to supplement his own work, or enough animals to necessitate leasing additional land. But even here there was marked gradation; not all *burgisi* were the same (W.F. Whyte, ''Sicilian Peasant Society,'' *American Anthropologist* 46 (1944): 65-74; also Chapman, *Milocca).*

10. Siverman, *Three Bells of Civilization,* 198-99.

11. Davis, *Land and Family in Pisticci.*

12. See S. Salomone-Marino, *Costumi e Usane dei Contadini di Sicilia, a Cura di Aurelio Rigoli* (Palermo, 1879/1968), 235-59; G. Pitrè, *Usi e Costumi, Credenze, e Pregiudizi del Popolo Siciliano* (Firenze, 1939), 2:27-39, 52-56; Whyte, ''Sicilian Peasant Society,'' 69-70

13. S. Leone, ''Costumi e Vita Sociale,'' in *Storia della Sicilia* (1978), 77:81-83; S.

Salomone-Marino, "Le Pompe Nuziali e il Corredo d'elle Donne Siciliane ne' Secoli XIV, XV e XVI," in *Archivio Storico Siciliano* 7 (1876):209 ff.

14. Salomone-Marino, *Costumi e Usanze dei Contadini;* Pitrè, *Usi e Costumi;* Whyte, "Sicilian Peasant Society."

15. P. Balsamo, *Memorie Inedite di Pubbli Economia ed Agricoltura* (Palermo; 1845), 1:127-8.

16. See D.E.C. Eversley, "The Home Market and Economic Growth in England, 1750-80," in *Land, Labour and Population in the Industrial Revolution,* E.L. Jones and G.E. Mingay, eds. (London, 1967), 212; N.B. Harte, "The Rise of Protection and the English Linen Trade, 1690-1790," in *Textile History and Economic History; Essays in Honor of Miss Julia de Lacy Mann,* N.B. Harte and K.G. Ponting, ed. (Manchester, 1973), 108. Decencies "for wear of the common people" proliferated in England nearly a century before Balsamo promoted their adoption in Sicily. In 1700, England imported just under 300,000 yards of Irish linen. By 1740, imports had reached 6.5 million yards. English linen industries grew rapidly in the same period, largely on the basis of imported Irish and Scottish thread. According to A.H. John, this is good evidence for expanded consumption of sheets and underwear among farmers, cottagers, and artisans, as well as the rich (John, "Agricultural Productivity and Economic Growth in England, 1700-1760," *Journal of Economic History* 25 [1965]: 19-34).

17. *Memorie Inediti,* 127.

18. Salomone-Marino, *Costumi e Usanze dei Contadini,* 253-57.

19. Pitrè, *Usi e Costumi* 2:27-8.

20. C. Wheeler, *The Development of Embroidery in America* (New York, 1921), 35.

21. R. Price and S. Price, "Noviazgo in an Andalusian Pueblo," *Southwestern Journal of Anthropology* 22 (1966): 312.

22. E.g., M. Stapley, *Popular Weaving and Embroidery in Spain* (New York, 1924), 56.

23. For a more complete description of the *civile* house, its contents and how they were made in the late nineteenth century, and especially of the spatial segregation of "culture" and "nature," see P. Schneider, "Class Formation and Material Culture in Nineteenth-Century Sicily," paper presented at the annual meeting of the American Anthropological Association, Los Angeles, 1978.

24. N. Elias, *The Civilizing Process; the History of Manners* (New York, 1939/1978), 143-153.

25. See Gabaccia, "Houses and People."

26. G. Cocchiara, *Il Folklore Siciliano,* vol. 1: *La Vita del Popolo Siciliano* (Palermo, 1957), 42-48; Pitrè, *La Famiglia, La Casa, la Vita del Popolo Siciliano* (Bologna, 1969), 55-63.

27. Cocchiara, *Il Folklore Siciliano* 1:38.

28. C. Bennetti-Ventura, *Trinee Donne Siciliane* (Milan, 1911).

29. For the proverb, see Pitrè, *Usi e Costumi,* 21-22. It has other tantalizing equations, which I am unsure how to interpret; for example, if the girl were spinning, it meant she would give birth to many children.

30. Bennetti-Ventura, *Trine e Donne Siciliane.*

31. Quoted in Pitrè, *Usi e Costumi,* 20.

32. *Il Folklore Siciliano* 1:36.

33. In 1866, a Palermo daily carried a brief article reporting damage to women's genitals from spending too many hours at an early model of the Singer. One operated this particular machine with an alternating, back and forth motion of the feet on a double treadle. We know from the history of later models that their worldwide distribution began in the late nineteenth century and it seems plausible that a few machines reached Villamaura to aid the *cucitrici* of the 1880s. I could not find any dates on the antique Singers which people still have, but they were said to be "in the family" for three generations.

34. See especially E. Sereni, *Il Capitalismo nelle Campagne (1860-1900)* [Torino, 1968], 3-41.

35. Not all of the new cloth was foreign, even though a great deal of it came from England. North Italian textile industries expanded with the unification of the national market during the 1860s, and especially under tariff protection 20 years later. Meanwhile, the Jacquard loom gave a few of Sicily's silk industries a new lease on life, one example being the Guli works in Palermo. With this loom, Guli could manufacture damasked cotton mattress covers that captured the *corredo* market in Southern Italy as well as Sicily, replacing the coarse, striped covers earlier woven at home (from an interview with descendants of the founder at the plant).

36. See D.P. Cole, *Nomads of the Nomads; the Al Murrah Bedouin of the Empty Quarter* (Chicago, 1975), 64, for a Bedouin parallel; also L.A. Hirschfeld "Cuna Aesthetics: a Quantitative Analysis," *Ethnology* 16 (1977):147-166.

37. A. Panzini, *Dizionario Moderno delle Parole Che Non Si Trovano nei Dizionari Comuni,* 9th ed. (Milano, 1956).

38. Vol. 9, 80.

39. G. Giacone, *Zabut; Notizie Storiche del Castello di Zabut e Suo Contiguo Casale-Oggi Comune di Sicilia* (Sciacca, 1932), 128.

40. See Pitrè, *La Famiglia, la Casa,* 143.

41. Cocchiara, *Il Folklore Siciliano* 1:49.

42. This is not to suggest, however, that the link between needlework and the demographic transition was universal. In Kutch and Saurashtra in India, where, incidentally, domestic embroidery also developed in the nineteenth century, it is the needles of older, married women that "throb with life" as they prepare embroidered trousseau for their soon to be child-bride daughters (J.N. Namavati, M.P. Vora, and M.A. Dhaky, *The Embroidery and Beadwork of Kutch and Saurashtra* (Baroda, 1966). And in Hungary, where "a girl of 14 is allowed to receive suitors" and one of 20 is "regarded as an old maid," the bride-to-be, young as she is, prepares her trousseau and an embroidered shirt for the bridegroom at the expense of learning how to bake bread, cook, and milk—skills crucial to her adult existence that she must then acquire from her mother-in-law. Her mother, however, "is expected to supply . . . an entire set of (handwoven) bed linen for everyday use," and an ornamental cover, if she can afford to make it (see E. Fel and T. Hofer, *Proper Peasants; Traditional Life in a Hungarian Village* (Chicago, 1969), 119-20, 130-33, 143). (Here too, dowry consisted largely of trousseau [ibid, 25]).

43. *Milocca,* 31-2, 54-60, 98.

44. See Pitrè, *La Famiglia, la Casa,* 34-6.

45. J.K. Campbell, *Honour, Family and Patronage; a Study of Institutions and Moral Values in a Greek Mountain Community* (Oxford, 1964), 302.

46. Pitkin, "Marital Property Considerations Among Peasants."

47. Chapman, *Milocca,* 36-41; E. Friedl, "The Position of Women: Appearance and Reality," *Anthropological Quarterly* 40 (1967): 97-109.

48. Quoted in Chapman, *Milocca,* 36.

49. E. Lefébure, *Embroidery and Lace: Their Manufacture and History From the Remotest Antiquity* (London, 1888), 128, 188-192; E. Ricci, *Ricami Italiani, Antichi e Moderni* (Firenze, 1958), 35-46.

50. V. Fagone, ed., *Arte Popolare e Artigianato in Sicilia; Repertorio dell'Artigianato Siciliano* (Caltanissetta/Roma:1966), 122-5.

51. Chapman, *Milocca,* 44.

52. Davis, *Land and Family,* 36.

53. See Davis, *Land and Family,* 173-4; also D.O. Hughes, "From Brideprice to Dowry in Mediterranean Europe," in this volume, p. 36.

54. Anonymous, *The Literary Digest,* 1921.

55. See S. Chojnacki, "Dowries and Kinsmen in Early Venice," *Journal of Interdisciplinary History* 4(1975): 571-600, R. Levi-Pisetzky, *Storia del Costume in Italia* (Milano, 1969), 5:942-6.

56. I am grateful to Ashraf Ghani for pointing out that the very large trousseaux of the *civile* class might have had an impact on the size of the market for embroidered whitewear.

57. See M.J. Herskovits, *Markets in Africa,* P. Bohannan and J. Dalton, eds. (Evanston, 1962), Preface.

58. Salomone-Marino, *Customi e Usanze dei Contadini,* 245.

59. The same ideological complex constrained men against expensive temptation, too, the temptation of alcohol in particular. Wives were explicitly concerned that male earnings, earmarked for dowry, not be dissipated in local taverns.

60. Pitrè, *Usi e Costumi* 2:63; *La Famiglia, La Casa,* 45-63.

61. Pitrè, *Usi e Costumi,* 63.

62. Chapman, *Milocca,* 104.

63. An important exception is the work of Jan de Vries ("Peasant Demand Patterns and Economic Development, 1550-1750," in *European Peasants and Their Markets,* W.N. Parker and E.L. Jones, eds. [Princeton, 1975]), which details a considerable expansion in the consumer behavior of Friesland peasants between 1550 and 1750 - probably two critical centuries for Europe as a whole. Increased production for market underlay the change and new items included a range of clothes and decencies, the famous Dutch window curtains, household furnishings, farm equipment, and so on. Of special note was an increase in luxury goods. Large farmers owned an average of 2.6 silver-buttoned waistcoats in the first half of the eighteenth century; 4.3 in the second. And they increasingly ate from tin dishes and porcelain rather than wood. But most important for our purposes was a rise in silver and gold objects within the home for as de Vries says, these were "not just consumer goods but also a store of value . . . a reasonably liquid form of wealth with an extremely long depreciation period." In the sixteenth century there were few such things, only rings, buttons, chains, and buckles, by the seventeenth century, women had silver waistbands with key chains, knife sheaths, and purses, all partly of silver, attached; and in the early eighteenth century, prosperous peasants owned gold rings, silver spoons, silver and gold buttons, beakers, cups, and mustard pots. An object called an oorijser, which bound women's hair, was of iron in the Middle Ages, silver by the late seventeenth century, and gold by the eighteenth. It also grew in width until by the second half of the 1700s, "it nearly covered the skull (pp. 222-24)."

64. D. Mack Smith, *A History of Sicily; Modern Sicily After 1715* (London: 1968), 406; S. Sonnino, *I Contadini in Sicilia* (Firenze, 1925), 219-31.

65. E.g., R. Giuffrida, "I Problemi della Circolazione Monetaria Siciliana dalla Fine del Settecento alla Prima Meta dell'Ottocento," in *Storia della Sicilia* (1978) 7:122.

66. Mack Smith, *Modern Sicily After 1715,* 383, 454-6.

67. L. Yang, *Money and Credit in China: A Short History* (Cambridge, Mass, 1952).

68. D.W. Ames, "The Use of a Transitional Cloth-Money Token Among the Wolof," *American Anthropologist 57* (1955): 1016-24.

69. Quoted in A. Dolby, *Church Vestments; Their Origin, Use and Ornament, Practically Illustrated* (London, 1868), 24-5.

70. P. Johnston, *The Byzantine Tradition in Church Embroidery* (London, 1967), 9-10. Also see A. Krsteva, *Macedonian Folk Embroidery* (Skopje, 1975); A.J.B. Wace, *Mediterranean and Near Eastern Embroideries,* from the collection of Mrs. F.H. Cook, vol. 1 (text), (London, 1935).

71. Johnston, *Byzantine Tradition in Church Embroidery,* 65.

72. M. Schuette and S. Müller-Christensen, "German and Italian Embroidery of the Middle Ages," *Craft Horizons* 24(1964): 50. Also see Ricci, *Ricami Italiani,* 30.

73. Wace, *Mediterranean and Near Eastern Embroideries,* 51-2.

74. Johnston, *Byzantine Tradition in Church Embroidery,* 10-23, 77.

75. Ibid., 65-71.

76. Lefébure, *Embroidery and Lace,* 41.

77. Ibid., 172; Ricci, *Ricami Italiani,* 42-6.

78. Dolby, Church Vestments, 13. Also M. Undi, *Hungarian Fancy Needlework and Weaving: The History of Hungarian Decorative Embroideries and Weavings, From the Time of the Occupation of Hungary by the Magyars until Today* (Budapest, n.d.).

79. Lefébure, *Embroidery and Lace,* 157.

80. Ibid., 163.

81. Recent accounts of this process suggest a continuum from situations where embroidery for the tourist market is occasional, and intended only to meet the most pressing needs for cash (Hirschfeld, "Cuna Aesthetics") to situations where commercialization has transformed the activity into a cottage industry (R. Waterbury and C. Turkenic, "Embroidery for Tourists: The Spontaneous Evolution of a Putting-Out System in a Mexican Peasant Community," paper presented at the annual meeting of the American Anthropological Association, Los Angeles, 1978).

Regarding the thorough-going sex segregation of the past, there were always exceptions. Chapman, for example, notes that "occasionally a man will boast proficiency in some feminine task . . . the men who go to prison sometimes learn weaving and embroidery, and their handiwork is displayed with pride when they send it home (*Milocca,* 33).

For Love or Money: The Marriage Strategies of Jews in Imperial Germany

Marion A. Kaplan

> A Roman woman once asked Rabbi Jose, "In how many days did the Holy One . . . create His world?" "In six days," he answered. "Then what has He been doing since . . . ?" "He sits and makes matches," came the response, "assigning this man to that woman, and this woman to that man." (*Midrash Rabbah,* Genesis, section 68)

The customs surrounding the arrangement of Jewish marriages in Imperial Germany reflected ancient Jewish traditions, but also mirrored prevailing practices among the German bourgeoisie. Jewish attitudes toward love, marriage, financial security and parental control were in many ways quite typical. A predominantly middle-class Jewry, like its Gentile counterparts in an industrializing capitalist economy, sought to concentrate capital through dowries and to create economic and social alliances through marriage. Jewish expectations and habit revealed the conflict between the commonplace reality of arranged marriages of convenience and the emerging ideal of romantic, companionate marriage. By the beginning of the twentieth century, Jews and other Germans increasingly acknowledged a more sentimental interpretation of the marital relationship. Yet, it was only after the First World War that the confluence of structural and post-war economic conditions—not least of which were the entry of middle-class women into the labor force and the damage to middle-class savings caused by the inflation—successfully challenged the control middle-class parents had over their children's decisions and permitted young people to "fall in love".

"For Love or Money: The Marriage Strategies of Jews in Imperial Germany," by Marion A. Kaplan is a revised version of a longer essay which appeared in The Leo Baeck Institute Yearbook XXVIII, 1983

The Jewish experience was also distinctive, shaped by the status, aspirations and fears of a minority. Jews differed from the majority in their emphasis on endogamy and their frank concern with financial security. As a distinct religious and ethnic group, Jews were committed to the perpetuation of the Jewish family as an indispensable social institution for maintaining their religion and community. As a minority in a society which increasingly practiced racial discrimination, most Jews sought endogamy and, in fact, had little other choice. Finally, as a group highly concentrated in business, economic interests markedly influenced their marriage decisions. Thus, a study of Jews will highlight the particular concerns of a minority as it typified socially prevalent attitudes towards "love or money".

The first section of this essay will describe how Jewish marriages were arranged and the relative importance of religious, financial and personal factors in these arrangements. The second will focus on Jewish and Gentile criticisms of the "dowry chase", particularly the widely shared perception that Jews were more interested in financially auspicious marriages than non-Jews. It will offer reasons for this perception, but will suggest that Jewish financial strategies were similar to those of Gentiles of their class. The third section of the essay will survey the more "modern" ways in which people married, including the infinite variety of arranged "coincidences" by which couples met and the small, but growing number of love matches. In sum, this study of Jewish marriage arrangements and dowries reflects upon the economic and social aspirations of Jews, the socialization and expectations of women and men, and the marriage patterns common among the commercial classes and the *Bildungsbürgertum* in Imperial Germany.

TO THE HIGHEST BIDDER: ARRANGED MARRIAGES AND DOWRIES, 1871-1918

The socialization and education of women in Imperial Germany had prepared most of them for, and limited them to, marriage. Marriage was a serious business, too serious to be left to the whims of the individuals involved. Among Jews, parents, family, friends and matchmakers served to find the appropriate partner for a young woman. Marriages were contracts between families: material factors were of primary importance.[1] This varied according to class, with the upper strata, where marriages involved substantial property transfers, exerting the greatest control over love and courtship behavior. Families saw their goal as providing young women with economic security and a socially acceptable role, that of wife. Women, in turn, had to provide for their own happiness, by controlling their behavior and emotions so as not to interfere with their status and duties.

Although new attitudes toward love as the foundation of marriage had received public attention in Germany with the development of the Romantic School of the early nineteenth century, it took over one hundred years for these ideas to become widely accepted. By the end of the nineteenth century, middle-class families began to pay lip service to notions of sentiment and love. As memoir literature and intermarriage statistics[2] imply, there were more opportunities for a minority of young people to respond to romance and more occasions when they announced their intentions to their parents. However, as we shall see, this was the exception rather than the rule. And, even then, couples sought parental consent and understood the importance of financial considerations. For the majority, those involved in arranged marriages, the tension between an impossible and irrelevant romantic ideal and a more practical reality, was resolved by covering up arrangements to look as though the partners had met by coincidence. When this was not possible, participants attempted to solve the contradictions between "love" and "marriage" by "falling in love" during the engagement or shortly after the wedding. The incongruity between ideal and reality could be found in the popular literature and social criticism of the era. In the cliché-ridden and popular books of Elise Polko (1863), German women read of conventional roles for women, of subservience to men, of motherhood and housewifery, only to be transported into the realm of "love at first sight". "When his eyes struck her, her soul underwent the most meaningful changes. . .and as the desired and feared hour neared, in which. . .the words 'I love you' fell. . .the golden doors of a new world opened."[3] The satirical weekly, *Simplicissimus,* debunked such romantic nonsense as a figment of bourgeois imagination and contrasted it with a reality which forced middle-class women into mercenary marriages: "The Chinese are certainly barbarous. . .they sell their girls openly in the marketplace!" a man informed a woman at a party. The woman replied, "Why isn't that awful! How long will it take them to learn to sell their girls in private, as we do?"[4]

For Jews, as for other bourgeois Germans, marriages of convenience (*Vernunftehen, Versorgungsehen)* were a commonplace throughout the period under study. Yet marriage patterns as well as attitudes towards marital partnership did not remain entirely static. A slow evolution from traditional attitudes prepared the way for the more modern courting and marriage patterns brought about by long-term structural changes as well as the First World War and post-war economic dislocations.

In order to analyze the various forms of marriage and the changes in marriage customs, we must define what is meant by "dowry", "trousseau", and "arranged marriage". For purposes of definition, a dowry *(Mitgift)* was a transfer of property to the bride from her family as she entered marriage. This property could consist of cash, real estate, jewels, stocks, or other transferable wealth. Dowries predominated among bourgeois and propertied peasant marriages in the period from 1870 until 1918.[5] Their persistence allowed a small middle class to accumulate capital by redistributing its savings among other members of its stratum, while those below—and often, above—scrambled for similar means of creating and perpetuating wealth. For women, the dowry weakened the social situation of the unmarried, particularly those in the lower ranks, while it continued to bolster the social status of a relatively small group of women of means by adding to their economic weight and, hence, familial status. Among the latter were most German-Jewish women, a result of the predominantly middle-class status of German Jews in Imperial Germany. For the minority of German-Jewish women, those too poor to accumulate capital, their work became their dowry.

Along with a dowry, German middle-class and propertied peasant women were expected to bring an extensive trousseau (*Aussteuer, Ausstattung)*into the marriage.[6] This often included linen, clothing, table ware, kitchen utensils and furniture. Among peasants, the trousseau, particularly the hand-embroidered linen, was of great importance: "when a young woman married, she often possessed far more linen than she needed for her household."[7] Families invited their neighbors in to examine the linen and needlework to everyone's delight and admiration.[8] The trousseau became the pride of middle-class *hohere Tochter* as well. Confined to the home after their meagre education, they stitched away the "waiting period", the time between graduation and marriage, on the linen and finery that would "last them a lifetime."[9] By the turn of the century, even this pastime became superfluous as more middle-class families bought extensive linen trousseaux in stores which began to specialize in these items.[10] As stores began to carry lines of trousseau furniture, costs mounted. The trousseau was as expensive as it was extensive: a bill could run from 2,000 to 3,000 M. for all necessary linen, kitchenware, and a bedroom suite. Another 2,500 to 3,000 M. would buy a dining room, living room and kitchen furniture.[11] In *Die Familie,* the conservative writer Wilhelm Riehl bemoaned the expansion of the trousseau in the mid- and late-nineteenth century. He complained that whereas the trousseau used to be made up of a few trusty old pieces of the family's furniture, it now had to be brand new.[12]

Equipped with a substantial dowry and trousseau, a young woman could expect to have her future, that is, her marriage, arranged for her. Formal, *arranged marriages,* with rare exception, were unions including dowries. They were unions involving a substantial exchange of wealth for security. While, as we shall see, a complex combination of age, status, looks, education, religiosity and geographical location was a factor in the equation, the primary transaction was one in which dowries and trousseaus were traded for a bridegroom's financial position. The partners met on the initiative of others for the express purpose of matrimony. In an arranged marriage, the union was determined far more by economic concerns than by personal inclinations. Although the prospective bride and groom were invariably asked if they found their intended partner suited to them, before the turn of the century it was the rare individual who answered in the negative: "That would have been a gross insult, for in truth one married. . .'into a family' " (Poznań, 1870).[13]

Such an officially arranged marriage must be distinguished from a relationship in which the couple met as a result of others' intervention, but where marriage was not the openly acknowledged goal. A marriage resulting from an informal or coincidental situation—although possibly foreseen by those involved—was not in a strict sense arranged. Although such a union proceeded within social and economic parameters which were consciously or unconsciously respected—often including dowry considerations—the couple involved took some initiative and expressed individual desires.

Before the 1870s, Jewish marriages had, with few exceptions, been arranged.[14] In her memoirs, Glückel von Hameln, born in 1646, described her own two arranged marriages as well as those of her twelve children, noting the significance of financial considerations. Families respected a "good name" and religiosity, but dowries (often for boys and girls) were essential. Money was the only insurance Jews had against political and social insecurity. Barely tolerated by local rulers, Jews paid extortionate sums for residential permits and the right to eke out an existence. Dowries enabled families to finance investments and extend the businesses which paid for limited tolerance. Also, dowries served as the basis for establishing a home and family. Partners who came from different cities, and sometimes, countries, did not see each other before the wedding, but that did not seem necessary to Glückel. She rested assured that "forty days before the birth of every child, a call goes forth in Heaven: 'Such-and-such a child shall be given the daughter of So-and-so.'"[15] If the financial negotiations for a proposed match did not work out, then it had not "found favor with God". If the couple married, then it had been foreordained. Marriage brokers took an active role in facilitating this predestined union. Their contacts reached across national boundaries, particularly when seeking matches for the wealthy. But, even the poorest could anticipate an arranged marriage, although this often took longer. If a young woman had no dowry, she waited until a wealthy person or a communal organization provided a modest gift. Throughout the seventeenth and eighteenth centuries, arranged marriages and the need for dowries remained much as in Glückel's day. However, the bride and bridegroom generally met each other before the wedding and parents respected strong dislikes despite the financial penalties for breaking an engagement.[16]

Even as reformers challenged Orthodox assumptions and rituals in the mid-nineteenth century, Orthodox traditions regarding marriage arrangements continued to be observed by Liberal families. In 1900, one young woman found it perfectly normal for her father to announce: "Put on a white dress, today you are getting engaged!"[17] Families took the lead in finding suitable partners for their eligible members and in working out the details of the engagement and marriage contracts. They did this as a family service and/or as a *Mizvah* (a good deed). Women used kin and friendship networks for informal brokering, and men conducted the financial discussions which preceded any formal encounter. Whereas prospective brides remained passive, often unaware of their family's project, grooms, particularly older ones, also took initiatives. And, parents or relatives often pressed young women into marrying. The Friedmann family serves to illustrate the typical arrangements of the era. In 1889, a young businessman sent his friend to Mr. Friedmann to arrange a marriage with Mr. Friedmann's nineteen-year-old daughter, Eugenie. She had never met the man, but had noticed him when buying in his shop. Her father told her that a wealthy businessman had asked for her hand. Father, grandmother, and several aunts urged her to accept. In 1894, her parents informed twenty-three-year-old Martha Friedmann that a young suitor (*Freier*) would come to visit her. The young couple met and agreed to marry on the spot. Financial arrangements had already been discussed prior to their meeting and the individuals approved of each other's appearance and manners. Beyond this, they knew nothing of each other, assuming only that each would fulfil well-defined roles and duties. The last two Friedmann daughters met their future husbands through the intercession of friends and distant relatives in 1903 and 1906.[18]

Parents frequently arranged marriages after making formal inquiries with respected families or after coincidentally meeting a prospective partner for one of their children. The future in-laws of Flora Goldschmidt encountered her on a train journey. Vaguely aware of her family's favorable status and position, they enjoyed her company and decided they would like her as a daughter-in-law. The groom's family asked their friend, Flora's uncle, to introduce the young people. The young man visited her home on 14th May 1872. They were engaged on 1st June.[19] It had been love at first sight, between in-laws and the bride. The future father-in-law of Jacob Rosenheim took a more formal approach. He wrote a letter to Rosenheim's parents asking if their twenty-seven-year-old son would marry his seventeen-year-old daughter. Both families had corresponded about Jewish and philanthropic concerns but did not know each other personally. The young Rosenheim was engaged to his bride several days after they met and married a few weeks later.[20] Rosenheim later became the founder of the Orthodox *Agudas Yisroel.* Whereas Liberal Jews permitted some individual initiatives, among the Orthodox strictly arranged marriages continued to be the rule throughout the Imperial period. According to one observer (born 1880), "in the Orthodox tradition, every girl was suited to every man. She had so little personality that she could adjust to every man."[21]

Brothers, particularly when they were their sisters' formal guardians, often arranged marriage partnerships. In 1862, a seventeen-year-old was talked into marriage by her brother who was also her guardian. She and her contemporaries considered seventeen to be a very young age, but she dutifully submitted.[22] Another brother persuaded his sister to marry by assuring her that if she consented "then it will be as if you have bought yourself life insurance."[23] Brothers drafted friends as well as casual acquaintances in their pursuit of partners for their sisters. Some of these marriages, in turn, provided business opportunities for the brothers.[24] Throughout the Imperial period, brothers placed matrimonial advertisements in newspapers for their sisters. "Seeking for my sister . . ." advertisements and initiatives may have been particularly numerous in a society in which responsibility for the family fell to the eldest male when both parents were deceased.[25] Furthermore, according to a Jewish source: "Brothers only married when their sisters had been settled. They were brought up to regard this as a necessary moral preliminary to their own marriages."[26] While this assertion remains to be proved, there is some statistical evidence to suggest that brothers might have postponed their marriages in order to contribute to their sisters' dowries and see them married off.[27] Thus, family members were actively involved in helping each other find appropriate partners, ones who would suit the personal and financial requirements of the individual and the family.[28]

Parents made use of professional, business and friendship networks when their familial contacts were limited. Jewish villagers in South and South-west Germany, for example, had many ties with other Jews across the borders in France, Switzerland and Belgium and used these connections when they sought likely mates for their relatives or friends.[29] Needless to say, such marriages furthered business, professional and social contacts as well. In 1870, the well-known Jewish historian, Heinrich Graetz, asked a former student, Joseph Perles, whom he also considered a friend, to find a suitable husband for his daughter, Flora. He suggested that Perles' wife be consulted, informed them that Flora would receive a 1,000 Thaler dowry, and noted that she did not want to marry a rabbi. With those conditions in mind, his friends were to find him a son-in-law.[30] Friends, thus, served important functions of information gathering, providing gossip and news about a potential spouse's reputation and income. At other times they helped with introductions, and still other times they introduced potential partners without having been asked to do so.

When the efforts of family, business contacts and friends failed to produce a marriage partner, a marriage broker (*Heiratsvermittler* or *shadkhan*) was hired. These brokers were professionals, male and female, specializing in a particular financial class and in certain districts. After a successful union, they were paid a percentage of the dowry.[31] In a letter to a Jewish father in 1873, one such broker offered his assistance in finding a partner among the wealthy Berlin bourgeoisie: "I know many Jewish families, for example, *Sanitätsrat* Hymann, Dr. Mendel, Dr. Jakobsohn . . . and many others. I have bankers, factory owners, doctors, lawyers, etc. . . ."[32] Brokers placed their own marriage advertisements in Jewish newspapers, or responded to those of individuals. Also, they were recommended by satisfied customers.[33] While most brokers provided detailed information on a family's history and fortune, detective services offered more sensitive information. They warned their target audiences: "Don't marry or become engaged before you know exact details about. . .the person, family, dowry, reputation, previous history. Discreet special information available."[34]

Urban Jews were by no means the only Jews who called upon the services of professionals. In 1871, 20% of all Jews lived in big cities, while by 1910 this figure had leaped to 58%.[35] Thus, originally a majority and then a large minority of Jews resided in small towns and rural areas. Scattered about small towns and villages at a time when Jews made up only 1% of Germany's population to begin with, provincial Jews found it difficult to meet suitable partners. This geographic hardship was worsened by economic and social mobility. Young men chose to migrate to larger urban centers to pursue more lucrative careers. They did this around the time they embarked on a career path, at precisely marrying age. Since Jewish men migrated in greater numbers than women, the latter had particular difficulty in finding Jewish mates in their home towns. Thus, rural Jews made substantial use of the broker. In rural Württemberg, for example, brokered marriages were the rule.[36] In Hesse, too, a memoir reveals: "Jewish marriages in the countryside (also in the city) were, as with the peasant population, not made in heaven."[37] Local Jewish teachers frequently served as marriage brokers, using networks of teachers in other villages and towns. This enabled them to earn an extra income to bolster their meager salaries. Fees usually depended on the amount of the dowry. Whereas all brokers knew the finances of their customers, teachers were often able to comment on the personalities of their former pupils as well. One teacher who was broker to many marriages in Baden around the turn of the century, passed on both of his professions to his son.[38] Despite their general usefulness, brokers were suspected for their mercenary motives and were not usually well respected, "but in families with many daughters and few contacts, one willingly let him in by the back door."[39]

Those who could not afford or mistrusted marriage brokers, whose connections did not provide sufficient choice, or who preferred to make their own arrangements placed advertisements in local Jewish newspapers. Mirroring similar phenomena in German local and regional newspapers, where marriage advertisements could be found to abound, the notices filled a role which had traditionally been the function of a community or social group. In fact, they attest to the rapid geographic mobility as well as the changing social positions and aspirations of individuals, many of whom were often isolated from communal and local roots and connections. Many Jewish newspapers reserved sections for those seeking marriage partners. Samples can provide an indication of the range of dowries and of their relative importance, although we cannot, of course, know if these advertisements resulted in a match. Various factors were enumerated in those placed by women's families, such as geographic location, age, appearance, education, health, previous marital status, ability to engage in paid labor (if the dowry was small), and, sometimes, religiosity (e.g., "pretty, educated girl, religious but not Orthodox . . .").[40] Money, however, was the most important factor. In 1912, the editor of a Berlin Jewish newspaper could still comment that in marriage advertisements "in the first place, the main thing, the dowry and then the accessory, the gracious bride, is examined. . ."[41]

A sample of Jewish newspaper advertisements from Berlin, Cologne, Frankfurt a. Main and Ansbach/Strassburg as well as memoirs and interviews offer some insights into the marriage market and the going rate for brides in Imperial Germany. To marry into the upper bourgeoisie in Berlin, for example, a woman had to possess substantial wealth and position. In 1904 a woman with 75,000 M. sought a lawyer, doctor or independent businessman. The woman was described as pretty and "from an excellent family."[42] Another that same year offered a dowry of 50,000 M. and "more later" for a doctor or lawyer.[43] The price for professionals probably rose in the first decades of the twentieth century, so that the family of another woman had to offer 100,000 M. for a Berlin dentist in 1920.[44] Assets were used to set up a home, expand a business or begin a professional practice. As late as the 1920s, the wealthy Berlin bourgeoisie still exchanged substantial dowries. "Married couples established themselves with a dowry," recalled one woman. Commenting on her sisters' marriages in 1920 and 1921, she observed: "You could almost buy people. If you had so much you could buy a doctor or a lawyer: or if you didn't have so much you might have to settle for a businessman." She saw no difference between the customs of her grandmother's generation—"sometimes the man married only the dowry"—and those of her own. She recalled her grandmother's constant admonition: "Love is nothing. You don't marry for love; you marry to have a nice home, you marry a man who is a decent person and that's the finish."[45]

Dowries were not confined to the *haute bourgeoisie,* although the custom may have continued longest in this class. The Jewish middle strata of well-to-do shopkeepers, trades- and business-people were equally dependent on financial arrangements. In Berlin, a woman with a dowry of 30,000 M. could hope to attract a partner with an income of about 10,000 M., the annual profit margin for a successful shopkeeper or businessman. However, the woman also had to possess other attributes. A thirty-four year old owner of a men's clothing shop sought a 30,000 M. dowry with a woman "no older than 23."[46] The family of one eligible young woman embellished her 30,000 M. dowry, by advertising her youth (20 years old), looks ("very pretty"), education and family reputation ("from distinguished Israelite family").[47] Thirty thousand Marks appears to have been the mean dowry advertised in Berlin. This figure would have been considered very high in a small town or village.

A less substantial dowry would attract a man of even more modest means. For 20,000 M., a Berlin woman could hope for a husband who would earn about 6,000 M. annually, the salary of a mid-level civil servant.[48] Women with from 8,000 to 10,000 Marks could expect suitors who were independent craftsmen or white-collar workers (*Angestellte).*[49] Anything less might attract an artisan, especially if the woman indicated that she was willing to work outside the home.[50] The lowest amount offered in Berlin papers was 5,000 M. in search of an artisan. One exception, a "simple and domestic" young woman with 2,000 M. sought an "elderly, well-situated gentleman."[51] At the bottom end of the dowry scale, it was more likely for intermarriages to occur: thus, the example of the daughter of a Jewish cattle dealer whose 4,000 M. dowry bought her a Catholic husband who was a butcher.[52] Jewish men preferred wealthier Jewish women, and since a "surplus" of women (*Frauenüberschuss)* existed in this period, some Jewish women had to look elsewhere for husbands. When Jewish women married Gentiles, their economic status and the lack of available Jewish partners were the main causes.[53] In fact, in general it was at the bottom end of the dowry scale where women were allowed to "fall in love", for the dictates of parents who could not offer dowries were not as compelling. And, despite grave reservations about intermarriage, some parents acquiesced in the notion that their penniless daughter had found someone to provide for her.

Although dowries were highest in Berlin, other large cities were not far behind. For example, in 1909 in Breslau, a couple matched the groom's "worth" of 13,333 M. (a one-third partnership in his family's business) with the woman's 15,000 M. (10,000 M. in cash and 5,000 M. worth of furniture).[54] In Cologne and Frankfurt, women with only 10,000 to 12,000 M. were clearly at a disadvantage. They might have to be willing to work outside the home or to marry older, less desirable men, even widowers.[55]

Outside the major cities, Jewish men and/or their families demanded relatively smaller sums. In 1903, a twenty-eight-year-old doctor from a "big city" in Silesia could require around 50,000 M. from a bride.[56] In 1914, a wealthy business man who lived in a small village expressed interest in a woman with money, but was willing to settle for no dowry at all.[57] Nevertheless, in the rural countryside, among peddlers, cattle and horse dealers, dowries were still essential in the vast majority of marriage transactions. Where cash was lacking, the bride's father could offer financially valuable substitutes. This was the case in Silesia, where one father-in-law gave the groom three districts in which he could have a monopoly of peddling rights, and in Bavaria where the father-in-law of a cattle dealer gave a house valued at 25,000 M.[58]

The importance of dowries was obvious to all. Sometimes, the dowry became the goal and the bride simply the means to the end. Advertisements such as: "Young man . . . in manufacturing . . . with 10,000 M., seeks to marry into business or similar branch . . .", or, even more directly: "Cutter wishes to marry into a business" were not infrequent.[59] It was, indeed, the strikingly rare advertisement which made no mention of a dowry. One such, placed in 1902 by a woman herself, rather than under the usual auspices of her parents or brother, ignored financial considerations entirely, noting:

". . . have not stood apart from the women's movement, would like very much to marry now, in order to achieve happiness through mutual work."[60] Such an advertisement, seeking an egalitarian relationship on a non-commercial basis stood in stark contrast to most others.

Dowries determined not only the partner and the life style a woman might expect, but also the geographic area in which she would settle. With a generous endowment, women could hope to remain in or move to attractive locations, usually cities. The fewer resources a woman had, the more likely it would be that she might have to move to a smaller town. In 1906, for example, a young woman with a substantial dowry of 30,000 M. could leave her tiny village (of 900 people) and "move up" to a small town where her marriage had been arranged to a man with a "solid middle-class income", a trader in vinegar and dyes. In 1910, a woman from Regensburg with only 12,000 M. at her disposal was forced to move to a tiny village. Her dowry could only interest a man of middling means in a less desirable location. It was commonly concluded that when a city woman moved into a village, it was due to a small dowry.[61] This "downward" geographical mobility was unique to brides: it was the price they paid to maintain their class position when dowries were inadequate. Men rarely moved from larger to smaller towns for any reason.[62] They either imported wives to their small towns or migrated to larger cities in search of better business and marriage opportunities. Conversely, while brides moved to smaller places, single Jewish women rarely moved to larger cities on their own. As a result, there were many more women than men of marriageable age in the small towns and villages. This probably caused an inflation in the size of dowries needed to lure a diminishing supply of men. It is also likely that many families decided to migrate to urban centers when it became clear that daughters could not find suitable partners in their home town. Thus, not only business, educational and cultural opportunities, but family marriage strategies as well, contributed to the lure of urban life for Jews.

Aside from money and geographical location, age played a significant role in a woman's ability to marry. Men demanded that brides be no older than twenty-five; some set the limit at twenty-three. According to contemporary studies, the average age of Berlin bourgeois Jewish brides in 1909 was twenty-two to twenty-three for those marrying academics and twenty-three to twenty-four for those marrying businessmen.[63] Poorer women were slightly older, but twenty-five was often considered "too old" for any woman. By that age, most women were considered "old maids" and had resigned themselves to a life of spinsterhood with its financial insecurity and low social status.[64]

The giving of dowries among Jewish families with some means was an almost universal phenomenon which declined only slowly in the 1920s.[65] Dowries were taken for granted not only for the financial security they promised, but also for the power and status they conferred on the wife and her family.[66] The dowry preserved women's status in marriage. It was a woman's only psychological counterpoint to total dependency on her husband. In the decades that followed their marriage in 1912, for example, the wife of a Jewish cattle dealer often reminded him of her large dowry. It was taken for granted that her property preserved a respected position for her.[67] Wives and their parents were mindful of their contributions to husbands' businesses or practices and did not hesitate to recall these details if husbands acted too proudly or if there were family quarrels. Similarly, a substantial dowry increased a bride's authority *vis à vis* her in-laws. And, of course, the dowry was also an economic counterpoint. It is still common today for women of that generation to remember the value of their own, their relatives' and friends' dowries. They insist that these sums were just as important a contribution to their marriages as were the husbands' earnings. Further, the dowry was the wife's only financial recourse were the marriage to fail. Although German law gave the husband the right to manage and use his wife's dowry, it was not his possession. In most cases, the dowry reverted to the woman if the marriage ended.[68] Thus, the remark of a young man about his sisters' marriages, "the economic base of marriage was highly valued by Jews," must be interpreted broadly.[69]

All participants understood that a family's prestige was at stake during dowry negotiations. For a bourgeois family, the dowry was a measure of its reputation. For the petty bourgeoisie, in particular, the dowry was a source of parental pride. Parents had often economized drastically in order to accumulate their daughters' dowries. The following exchange from the novel *Moritzchens Tagebuch* (1908) illustrates this. Moritzchen and his childhood sweetheart had agreed to marry. Just before the wedding, the bride's father, a man of humble means, reproached the groom for not inquiring about the dowry. "Am I marrying Rahel or the dowry?" asked the groom.

The father replied angrily that he had not scrimped his whole life long to be outdone by his son-in-law.[70]

By the time *Moritzchen* was published, it was possible for such informal financial understandings, particularly those involving smaller amounts, to occur. In prior decades, however, parents engaged in formal negotiations; witnesses and notaries attended the writing of the contract. A typical marriage contract of the 1870s stipulated: the exact amount of the bride's dowry and a description of the trousseau; the dates when these were supposed to be delivered; the right of the bride's family to the dowry and her portion of the wedding gifts if she died childless within the first two years of marriage; the bride's rights if the groom died childless within the first two years; and the bride's right to her dowry, trousseau and wedding gifts in case of a divorce in which she was blameless. The groom usually renounced any further demands on the bride's family and promised to sign a formal receipt when the dowry and trousseau were delivered to him.[71] Sometimes the contacts included agreements between parents and children, such as one which promised 30,000 M. with the understanding that this was part of the daughter's inheritance. An arrangement between the groom and his business partners, providing for his widow's participation in the business, might also appear in a contract. Further, the groom could free his wife from the ritual of *Chalizah* (the law by which a childless widow had to marry her brother-in-law), by stating that he would give her a letter from his brother freeing her to marry whomever she chose if she became widowed.[72] Although most documents contained the individuals' promises to "remain true in marriage", to remain wedded for the length of their lives, or to engage in "mutually respectful treatment", and some even spoke of love, they were stamped by a notary and signed by two to four official witnesses.[73] Begun with an invocation to God, they ended as a legal business document.

It is unclear when these formally notarized statements began to be replaced by a handshake. In the 1880s, some parents accepted verbal commitments in front of witnesses.[74] By the mid-1890s, other families still demanded legal documents. However, in 1895, the groom's side of a 25,000 M. negotiation "took this as a vote of no confidence, but consented."[75] Most likely, the formal contracts lasted longest where the greatest property was involved. The extent of the negotiations which preceded the legal transactions is also unclear from the available literature. Probably by the end of the Imperial era, as a result of the further embourgoisement of German Jews and their acculturation to German styles of behavior, real bargaining and negotiating gave way to general agreement regarding a sum understood by both families to be socially acceptable.

Since dowries were essential to most Jewish marriages in Imperial Germany, parents, relatives and the Jewish community tried to ensure that young women might have at least modest means at their disposal when they reached adulthood. In some cases, middle-class parents bought dowry insurance which matured when girls reached the age of eighteen.[76] Wealthy relatives might be found to provide a sum if parents could not.[77] Jewish dowry clubs, too, donated funds to needy brides. Giving gifts to poor brides was a holy duty among the ancient Hebrews and medieval Jews. This custom was reinforced by a European (Christian) tradition harking back to the fourteenth century, in which public and private charities dowered the poor.[78] The dowering of brides was written into Jewish law. For example, in 1726, the Hamburg Jewish community stipulated that public collections could be scheduled to assist needy young women. Financial aid for prospective brides took precedence over most forms of charity.[79] By the nineteenth century, dowry-giving was most often organized by women's societies or by wealthy families. One such family, for example, maintained a book with the names of all the brides to whom it gave donations from 1810 to 1914.[80] Traditional women's charities as well as more modern ones focused on the needs of poor brides. The ubiquity and longevity of these charities—for example, the *Brautausstattung Stiftung* in Hamburg functioned from 1814 until 1913 and the *Israelitischer Brautausstattung Verein von 1840* (later the *Isr. Mitgift Verein),* also in Hamburg, lasted from 1840 to 1934—and the creation of new dowry clubs in the Imperial era[81] testified to their continued and renewed importance despite their modest donations.[82]

Women without recourse to any financial assistance might have one last opportunity to save themselves from spinsterhood. They could marry a widower, widely acknowledged to be a less than optimal match. Generally, widowers were a great deal older than their brides (and this in an era when a five- to seven-year age gap was considered normal). Often, they had children and were seeking mothers and housekeepers for them. Left with four children when his wife died in 1890, one man remarried within a year. When his second wife died in 1901, leaving him with nine children, he again remarried within the year.[83] In order to avoid the necessity of such a match, one brother married his sister off at twenty-one, afraid that if she were much older she would be forced to marry a widower.[84]

As women reached their late twenties, it was clear to outsiders that their chances were becoming more and more limited. People assumed that had they had money, they would have been married off. Not only were they aging, but they were also poor. One woman married a widower whose first wife had referred to her as one of those "*Mädchen* . . . who were waiting for the deaths of women in order to marry widowers."[85] To marry off women in danger of being "left behind" and to help widowers in their endeavors, the prescriptive literature of the period, particularly short stories written for Jewish family magazines, encouraged such marriages of convenience. Typical of this genre was the fate of the young governess who married the rich, old widower with children and lived happily ever after, "it is better . . . to face reality . . . ideals don't bring much."[86]

A more risky venture to avoid spinsterhood was emigration. Initiated by only a few, some women emigrated as a result of a marriage proposal, others in pursuit of marriage possibilities. "Generally, only poor girls accepted American marriage proposals."[87] Even without proposals, some families found themselves desperate enough to send daughters abroad to make their own way. In the 1890s, three daughters from a village family of nine children fled to the U.S. rather than remain single in Germany. In 1900, when the father of ten children could not afford a dowry for two of his five daughters, they also emigrated to the U.S. in hope of finding work and marriage there.[88]

We have seen the extraordinary importance attached to marriage decisions among the Jewish bourgeoisie in Imperial Germany. Marriages, arranged for the most part, were economic transactions intended to provide both partners with reciprocal benefits. They were also social contracts intended to reproduce the Jewish family and maintain the Jewish community. An elaborate network of parents, relatives, friends, associates, marriage brokers, insurance and charity organizations stood ready to facilitate and control marriages in order to avoid unfavorable alliances, emigration, or spinsterhood. Brides remained primarily passive, part of—but not always the most significant part of—the traffic in dowries. In a period of rapid capital accumulation the interdependence of the traditional gender system with the economic system gave a preeminence to dowries.

This would be challenged only later, by women's own careers and incomes as well as by structural and cyclical economic developments.

THE DOWRY CHASE: CRITICAL PERSPECTIVES

Although financial prerequisites for marriage were universally taken for granted, attacks upon the commercialization of marriage proliferated. Dowries were the object of persistent and serious criticism within the Jewish community. Many Jews criticised the questionable ethics involved in marrying money, they worried that marriages were being postponed in order to accumulate adequate or grandiose dowries, they feared that later marriages would produce fewer offspring for the Jewish community, and they were concerned that Jews were not living up to German norms. Also, they were anxious that Jewish women were being "left behind,"[89] a result of male migration, emigration, and intermarriage as well as the pursuit of dowries. As early as 1849, one could read in the broadly circulated *Allgemeine Zeitung des Judentums,* a critique of money marriages. The newspaper suggested (as did feminists then and later) that Jewish women learn a trade or the skills with which to contribute towards a family's existence. In that way, love and not money could be the deciding factor.

The journal located the problem among the "numerically preponderant middle class," not among the Jewish poor. Aware that Jews had been severely circumscribed to fields of business and commerce and that their recent emancipation from economic strictures would take years to realize, the *Allgemeine* acknowledged the desire of most young men to combine a favorable financial marriage settlement with the establishment of an independent enterprise. However, it urged Jews to recognize that a woman who could help in the business, or who could do without servants at home, would be just as useful as a young heiress, the more so, since a badly invested dowry could be lost forever. The newspaper chided parents that women's education was faulty: piano playing, singing and dancing were hardly as useful as being able to support themselves.

The *Allgemeine* concluded by placing the blame squarely on the woman's side. It ignored the desire of a newly-rich bourgeoisie to display its wealth by the leisure of its women and argued that men's demands could not change until young women had a more practical education.[90]

Orthodox spokesmen were also aware of the deleterious effects of dowry-centered marriages. In 1895, an editorial in the Orthodox family weekly, *Die Laubhütte,* worried about dowry inflation and predicted that middle-class women would soon be unable to buy husbands. Culpability rested once again with women: the journal censured girls who wanted luxurious life styles. Men simply could not afford to marry such wives without huge dowries. Echoing male complaints which can be traced as far back as the Renaissance, the *Laubhütte* also repeated age-old solutions: women had to lower their expectations.[91]

A generation later, in 1919, a letter to the *Israelitisches Familienblatt,* reiterated earlier concerns. The correspondent bemoaned the "tendency, among us Jews, to put the dowry in first place in the choice of a wife". The letter suggested that the situation could be improved if academically-trained men, that is, doctors or lawyers, married for idealistic rather than mercenary reasons. Businessmen, of course, needed dowries to invest in their businesses. Hence, even those who spoke out against marriages for money bowed to their "necessity" in most cases.[92] Jewish feminists, who denounced the "dowry chase," had no immediate solutions either. Beyond demanding economic independence for future generations of women, they could only criticize the "dowry chase", which was "not limited to Jewish circles."[93]

The tensions between the ideal of a companionate, "love" marriage and the financial realities of a "responsible" money marriage were often played out in literature. Jewish writers assailed the "Jewish" proclivity to emphasize dowries, although money marriages were not at all unique to Jewish circles. Jewish literature was replete with tales of and attacks upon arranged, money marriages. In a series of Jewish joke books published in the 1860s and 1870s, for example, the jokes and satires both reflected and criticized the pursuit of financial gain via marriage.[94] Arranged marriages between the children of business associates were held up to ridicule. In a series of satirical letters, grain merchants discussed business and the possible union of their offspring. In the spirit of their dickering over the prices of wheat and rye, they wrangled with each other over the size of the dowry. The engagement was announced twenty-five days after the start of the grain negotiations.[95]

In *Jettchen Gebert,* published in 1906 and one of the most popular novels of German-Jewish life, Georg Hermann dramatized the dilemma of a marriage of convenience. The heroine agreed to marry a man she did not love, although she was infatuated with another. She went through with the wedding, but then ran away and found refuge with her uncle. In a follow-up story (*Henriette Jacoby,* 1915), her aunt, a member of the older generation, tried to talk sense into her by explaining that marriage was, after all, only security:

> You have to try to get used to each other. If divorce were as easy as weddings, no marriage would last longer than a half year. . .my child. . .I don't understand you. What do you want from men? They're all alike after all.[96]

Both tales contained mixed messages. Hermann acknowledged love and woman's right to make a decision regarding marriage. Jettchen was "encouraged", though never overtly forced, to marry. Her divorce was supported, if reluctantly, by her family. Yet, Jettchen's romantic feelings were shown to be fleeting and had disastrous consequences. As a result of her escapades, the object of her affection was dismissed from the civil service. Her family was forced to pay her husband for his consent to the divorce, and Jettchen fell in love with yet another man. *Jettchen Gebert* went into its ninetieth reprinting in 1920 with many of its themes still of current interest.

An example of a less ambivalent literary treatment of the subject can be found in *Moritzchens Tagebuch* by Karl Ettlinger. Written in 1908, the book clearly advocated love over money. Moritzchen, an efficient and skillful salesman, attracted the attention of his employer. The latter tried to tie Moritzchen to his business by offering him his daughter and 40,000 to 50,000 Marks. When Moritzchen explained that he was already engaged, the employer simply raised the bid to a partnership in the business.[97] The crassest characters of all appeared in Artur Landsberger's *Millionäre* (1913), a critique of the Berlin-Jewish *nouveaux riches.* In danger of being publicly exposed as a swindler, a millionaire agreed to give his daughter as booty to his blackmailer.[98] Landsberger also reminded Jewish parvenus that their intermarriages with the nobility did not indicate their acceptance: his nobleman pursued rich Jewish heiresses in alphabetical order.

The self-criticism of German Jews was matched, if not exceeded, by the comments of non-Jews.[99] The latter complained that Jews extended "business-as-usual" into the arena of "love" and claimed that this was a peculiarly "Jewish" trait. In Poznań, for example, a county court judge commented (around 1905) to a Jewish *Landgerichtsrat,* "Jewish families are very strict in seeing that the dowry is paid out before the marriage. I have seen the wedding buffet cleared away, because the dowry had not been paid first."[100] In the countryside, peasants observed that Jews "traded their daughters like cattle. Marriage [was] more a thing of the money pouch than of the heart. Often it seemed like the cattle trade."[101] *Simplicissimus* also delighted in debunking the marriages of wealthy Jewish women with impoverished aristocrats. While Junkers looked none too good in these cartoons, Jewish wealth and Jewish arranged marriages for social prestige were held up to universal scorn.[102] It seemed to be particularly distasteful when Jewish money achieved social "respectability" by marrying into the nobility.

Whereas *Simplicissimus* spotlighted a statistically insignificant but, for some, socially unsettling, phenomenon, the country court judge and many peasants took the economics of marriage very seriously. Most probably, they had been married according to financial requirements themselves. Although arranged marriages for economic motives were commonplace among the German bourgeoisie and prevalent among the upper strata of peasants, it was Jews who were attacked for practices considered cynical and material, anachronistic and "foreign". Careful to shield their own marital motives, these commentators vented their hostility toward Jews as business people, middle men, "exploiters," or social climbers.

These observations lead to the difficult question of how representative such marriages were among Gentile Germans, and to its corollary: to what extent had Jewish practices remained distinct from those of their neighbors and to what extent had Jews merely maintained the norms of their class and region? Further, they suggest an inquiry into the discourse surrounding Jewish marriage strategies. Whether or not Jews were actually involved in more money marriages than non-Jews, why were they singled out with vehemence as flagrant offenders?

Although a comprehensive study of German marriage customs has yet to be written, we do know that in the early nineteenth century marriages among the peasantry and bourgeoisie were customarily arranged. Families depended on kin and friends to introduce young people to each other. When these failed, they also used more "modern" forms to arrange marriages, such as newspaper columns and brokers. The first marriage newspapers (*Heiratszeitungen*) appeared at the beginning of the century. One such journal, the *Hei-*

ratstempel included advertisements for inheritances and dowries. A man "with good prospects" sought a woman with 1,500 Thalers.[103] By the end of the century, notices still appeared in the personal columns, located directly after the "business opportunities" and "jobs wanted" sections of general newspapers. As late as 1914, one man sought a business venture, preferring a marriage into a business; another demanded a slim, cheerful woman with 200,000 M.; and still another described his income and university degree, asking for a photograph and the financial résumé of any respondents.[104] Notices placed by the families of women immediately referred to their dowries: "Christian woman with. . .300,000 M.", or "landowner's daughter with 300,000 M."[105] If she had nothing to offer, a woman might express her modest desires: "my own hearth at the side of an honored and beloved husband."[106] The non-Jewish bourgeoisie made use of brokers and detectives as well. The former often specialized in a particular group, such as industrialists, government officials, or spa visitors, and the latter promised strictest discretion in their pursuit of dowry and personal information.[107] In the midst of these traditional assumptions and institutions, a reader could encounter the contradictions provoked by modern expectations: the mother of an army officer, for example, sought a Protestant woman of "appropriate" status for a marriage of affection (*Neigungsheirat)*with her son.[108]

The German middle class was not alone in arranging its marriages. Well into the twentieth century, propertied peasants, for the most part, insisted on arrangements which included dowries. In the popular novel *Barfüssele* (1862, reprinted through 1912), Berthold Auerbach's peasant heroine and all who knew her believed she could never marry because she had no dowry. Poetic license alone brought her to the altar.[109] The characters as well as the readers understood how lucky she had been. Contemporary observers stressed the importance of dowry issues for north German peasants in the mid- and late nineteenth century.[110] Recent demographic surveys corroborate the importance of dowries for the Bavarian peasantry as well.[111] In Hesse, too, current studies testify to the continued significance of dowries in the 1920s. Well-to-do horse farmers used matchmakers who were usually cattle or grain dealers, people "who got around in the district and [were] familiar with the financial and social situation of the various farms with sons and daughters of marriageable age. . . . Material factors were to the fore." As with their Jewish neighbors, these, too, marriages were contracts between households.[112] Love matches were more common among the poorer cow farmers and most common among the impecunious goat farmers.

Peasants were not the only rural residents to seek arranged marriages. Village teachers, whose incomes were low, but who hoped to maintain a status appropriate to that of a *Beamter* (tenured civil servant) sought "suitable" wives. In the 1880's, the Jewish teacher in a small Hessian village helped to arrange the marriage of his Protestant friend, the village elementary school teacher. Offering to find his friend "a rich woman. . .so that the peasants will respect you," the Jewish man eventually came up with a woman who was "educated, [had] good manners and [was] a good cook."[113] In the countryside, then, most wealthy peasants as well as the rural bourgeoisie continued to arrange marriages with dowries, while less propertied residents allowed children to meet each other at religious festivals, village occasions (*Spinnstuben,* sporting events, harvests) and holidays. All such meetings took place in public, for "social control was vital and choosing one's partner for life was a public process."[114] Even though these marriages may not have been formally arranged, they were still unlikely to take place if parents disapproved. Non-arranged, but "approved" love matches prevailed among the poorest rural population.

Rural Jews lived in a group apart. Although they maintained social and business relations with their neighbors, they remained separate from non-Jews as a result of their religion, class and life style.[115] Their business needs and desire for endogamy contributed to the preservation of arranged money marriages long after the rural poor began to exert independent choice. Small shopkeepers, merchants, grain and cattle dealers, Jews tended to approximate bourgeois mores rather than adopt peasant customs. Dowries provided the necessary capital with which young men furthered their business interests and supported new families. Also, on the whole, rural Jews were religious. They sought endogamy at all costs and were likely to arrange a marriage before an offspring developed her or his own tastes. Since, as noted earlier, rural areas offered an increasingly limited pool of Jewish men, it was all the more urgent to arrange alliances with Jews from outside the village.[116] Arranged marriages prevailed where religiously- and class- appropriate mates were in shortest supply, diminishing in frequency in cities with large Jewish populations where religious and class endogamy could be achieved without formal arrangements. In an era of greater freedom of choice for some rural residents, Jews were conspicuous in their heavy reliance on arrangements.

So striking a difference between Jewish and Gentile marriage practices was not apparent in the cities. In the 1860's British observers noted that they had never heard of a single love match in the German city in which they lived and that in the provinces the dowry of every girl was known to the last penny.[117] At least through the turn of the century, most urban bourgeois parents attempted to arrange, formally or informally, the financially satisfactory marriages of their offspring. Although notions of "love" began to enter the equation, few marriages were calculated on this alone. In Hamburg in 1903, the eighteen year old Karen Horney confided to her diary: "It is bad. . .when one comes to know how few marriages are really good ones. . .Will it ever change? . . . . Perhaps even the next generation. . .will already be stronger than we are because more of them stem from a union of love."[118]

Love notwithstanding, novels, marriage ads and social histories of bourgeois marriages attest not only to the importance of financially based marriages in Imperial Germany, but to the *growing* importance of dowries in the prosperous years after 1890. In the period between 1860 and 1890, most academically educated *Beamten* had jealously guarded their *Stand* (estate), their social status and privilege. In a period of rapid commercial and industrial development, their allegiances shifted: they dropped the static concept of *Stand* in favor of the class privilege and status conferred by capitalism. They married the daughters of businessmen. In a study of Westphalia, for example, an author notes: "The attempt to achieve property via marriage was dominant.[119] Still convinced of their own importance, *Beamten,* nevertheless, appeared more willing to trade their status for their brides' wealth to assure themselves a standard of living beyond their own small salaries and in line with their expectations of their positions. Any luxury in the lifestyle of a civil servant, such as building his own home or buying property, could be attributed to his wife's dowry.[120]

Much like their counterparts in the civil service, those in the liberal professions such as doctors, lawyers, notaries and pharmacists also depended on their wives' dowries. They preferred the daughters of industrialists and businessmen in order to secure their incomes. The dowry supported comfort and luxury while the husband's salary paid for the rent, food and servants.[121] These men also wedded their education and status to the wealth of their wives' families. In turn, parents became even more conscious of the need to save up for their daughters' dowries as opportunities to "marry up" increased.[122] The stakes were high. Daughters without large dowries found no partners willing to marry them. Those single women who first entered the civil service in 1882 as ticket clerks and telegraph operators for the railways were from middle-class families. They had some education, but neither the "obligatory dowry" nor parents with the means to provide for them.[123] Dowries—or the lack of them—were the cause of women's upward or downward social and economic mobility. Neither class, status, education nor personal traits could compensate for a lost dowry. Dowries were among the most salient factors in the lives of all German bourgeois women at least until the First World War.[124]

We have noted the prevalence of money marriages among propertied Christians and Jews up to the war. The urban and rural bourgeoisie as well as propertied peasantry arranged financially appropriate marriages for their children. Jewish financial strategies were similar to those of Gentiles of their class. However, they stood out for several reasons. The Jewish economic profile was highly skewed, Jews being a predominantly commercial middle class. Jewish practice stood in sharp contrast to that of the urban working class and most of the rural population. Also, as a result of their minority position and geographic dispersion, Jews may have engaged in more energetic forms of marriage brokerage than Gentiles of their class or region. Still, Jewish customs were far from unique. In fact, they typified bourgeois expectations and behavior. Why then, were Jewish arranged marriages condemned and Jewish dowries disdained?

Dowries are generally more important where wealth and status are not balanced.[125] In a rapidly industrializing capitalist economy, a great deal of status anxiety and tension surrounding economic dislocation found poignant expression in complaints about dowries and marriages arranged for financial mobility. While Gentile and Jewish bourgeois economic fortunes rose, those below them suffered economic disruption and psychic and social dislocation. Above them, a "greedy warrior-agrarian class," which denied the importance of money and longed for an imaginary past where honor determined one's social position, faced economic decline.[126] The traditional concept of *Stand* had been undermined by achievement *(Leistung)* and its embodiment, wealth: the size of the dowry, not only the group to which one was born, determined one's place in society.[127] Those who watched their status slip as well as those with rising expectations found the dowry dilemma particularly painful, because it so clearly symbolized the power of money over the lives of their children and the future of their families.

Jewish financial prowess—the result of Gentile discrimination and acquired skills—appeared particularly irksome to those who saw their own positions slipping or whose daughters could not marry. In an era shaken by the crash of 1873 and increasingly anxious over the deficiencies of capitalism and liberalism—both associated in the popular mind with Jews—much of the disparagement of Jewish marriage strategies may be attributed to growing antisemitism. Whereas it is clear that the wealth of the industrial and commercial bourgeoisie in general, not of Jews in particular, undermined traditional social relations, the "pariah capitalists" of a previous era were excoriated.[128]

Ironically, antisemitism was also the cause of the overtly economic orientation of German Jews towards marriage. The Gentile middle class, aping the nobility's hypocritic contempt of money, avoided talk of what it felt to be base, material motives by stressing the social status a marriage could offer. Jews could partake of no such camouflage. While Gentile families could, indeed, use dowries to cement new social alliances, Jews were ostracized from "good society." For the most part unable and unwilling to marry into the Gentile elite, Jews concentrated on consolidating their financial worth by marrying into their own wealthier strata. Jews were not as likely—nor could they afford—to deny the significance of financial arrangements.[129] For them, money traditionally signified security in a hostile environment. Lucrative marriages meant increased security for their children. Thus, while all bourgeois parents attempted to arrange financially auspicious marriages, Jews were more overt and Gentiles more covert in their acknowledgement of this issue.

In an age which was beginning to reassess the terms of marriage, a bourgeoisie loath to criticize its own assumptions and practices regarding marriage castigated Jews as the incarnation of marriage-as-business. Only through wealth could the industrial and commercial bourgeoisie, vilified as vulgar upstarts by those they admired, achieve the higher status they sought. Caught between the desire for respectability and their embarrassment at their mean materialism, they insisted on the superiority of love or social status marriages,[130] they denied the extent to which their dowries bought status, and they denigrated Jews who avowed the consequence of money. Peasants, too, both those for whom such marriages may have begun to lose their economic rationale as well as those who continued to pursue financial goals, deprecated Jews as the beneficiaries of such relationships. Jews seemed as much the issue as the customs surrounding their marriages. That Jews were singled out disparagingly as particularly adept at arranging marriages for money in a society in which dowries were part of an old Gentile and Jewish tradition and in which the vast majority of the middle classes and propertied peasantry aspired to financial advancement through marriage, may tell us more about rising antisemitism than about a particularly "Jewish" proclivity. It elucidates the anxieties, jealousies and disdain of Germans caught first in a severe Depression and then in a period of phenomenal growth toward the real and imagined successes of a predominantly middle class Jewry and toward the real and imagined importance of money to these outsiders. In the discourse surrounding dowries and arranged marriages, one can discern the conjunction of anticapitalism and antisemitism.

"MODERN" MARRIAGES IN IMPERIAL GERMANY

Historians have recently suggested that changes in marriage patterns took place in the nineteenth century, including greater freedom in the choice of marital partners, less parental control over marriages, and a more companionate relationship within marriage. Families developed, based on sentiment, affection and free choice rather than on obligation or material considerations. Many bourgeois Jewish families no longer met or married in the strictly traditional mode, but they were not in the *avant-garde* of the "free choice" group either. Whereas traditional Judaism recognized the concept of a "successful marriage," not a "happy" one (success being dependent upon a "normal" sex life and a harmonious, as opposed to quarrelsome, relationship),[131] Jews in Imperial Germany entered a transitional stage. Although economic and social reality took precedence (the practical basis for a "successful" marriage), there was also a growing awareness of the social discourse concerning sentiment and affection (the basis for a "happy" relationship). Between 1870 and 1900, expressions of affection between partners gradually became common. Even though marriage was still a duty, a young couple was permitted, in fact, encouraged, to "fall in love." Elders had selected the eligible mate and, under their supervision, the betrothed could engage in courting behavior. For those who lived far apart, this might include an extensive correspondence (the *Brautbriefe)* in which partners discussed their likes and dislikes, their observations and opinions. For those within traveling distance, this usually involved chaperoned visits by the groom, public promenades walking "arm-in-arm" (a sign to the community that they were engaged)[132] and other formal family and community occasions. A complicated interaction between what was supposed to happen (that is, "love") and what was actually happening (that is, anticipation of marriage, common curiosity, and an attempt to be cooperative and pleasing), took place. Social expectations brought about predictable results in some cases: letters between fiancés frequently announced their "love" of each other, although they had barely met. Also, romantic notions may have been easier to conjure up when partners hardly knew each other.

Conscious of the growing contradictions between social ideology and social reality, some parents "covered up" traditional, arranged marriages. Others arranged circumstances where certain young people could meet each other. Still others allowed their children to fall in love without any familial control over the immediate situation. By the turn of the century, but in some cases even earlier, Jewish families began to pay lip service to "coincidence" or to camouflage actual arrangements in order to accommodate to modern sensibilities and protect the feelings of the young couple. Probably, Jews also attempted to adapt to what they considered the changing norms of the era as a result of their own desire to acculturate and in order to avoid criticism by Gentiles and antisemites. Spontaneity and coincidence developed into a fine art in the cities (where more opportunities for spontaneity existed) and among the non-Orthodox. Memoir and popular literature described both the arrangements and the pretense of spontaneity—ritual spontaneity—that had to be observed.[133] One father contrived to have a distant relative arrange the marriage of his daughter. The couple met "coincidentally" at a flower show where the young man was introduced as a business acquaintance of the father.[134] Some participants either never discovered that their meetings had been arranged or never admitted it. In Breslau in 1911, for example, the father of a thirty year-old widower hired a marriage broker for his son. The woman found an appropriate partner and arranged, through mutual associates, for the young couple to meet with friends at a cafe. Many years later, a close relative wrote: "To this day A and E. . .do not know they were brought together by a marriage broker."[135]

In the countryside, where arranged marriages became ever more necessary as Jews migrated to urban regions, such marriages began to be covered up too, but later. During the prewar years, families would often arrange marriages by orchestrating a chaperoned meeting of the intended couple. This took place at a restaurant, at a friend's home, or at markets and fairs (including horse markets). If the young people liked each other, negotiations followed. If an engagement was announced: "One heard everywhere that the young people had met there or there by 'coincidence' and that it was a real love match."[136] "The Love Match," a poem in a book of Jewish humor, gave a similar account: at a wedding reception an uncle made a toast to "love," while the marriage broker reflected on the difficulties of arranging this match.[137] Cover-ups could cause embarrassing situations, such as the one in Poznań, where the rabbi's wedding speech about the young "love match" he was sanctifying caused general hilarity in the audience.[138]

Alongside the formal arrangement of coincidences, a more modern pattern emerged around the turn of the century. It became more common for parents to influence the informal social contacts of their children so that they would meet only suitable peers.[139] One strategy was to plan propitious circumstances, such as vacations, for meeting eligible partners. Many a marriageable young person met a future spouse on a family vacation at a resort selected by the parents. Such was the case for one couple who "fell in love at first sight" at a mountain hotel in 1898. Their courtship was a peculiar, but not unrepresentative, mixture of traditional and modern forms. Her interest had been aroused by physical attraction: "his brown eyes have bewitched me," she told her sister. His feelings must have been reciprocal, for without exchanging so much as one word with his future wife, he discussed his intentions with her mother. The "bride" was dismayed at his behavior—"we were much too modern [for that]"—but waited until he visited her at home, again with only her mother's permission.[140] The *Kur,* a spa for recuperation or vacation, was another very popular place for meeting a future spouse. Ostensibly for one's health and one's nerves, spas in Germany, France and England provided real antidotes to spinsterhood.[141] Needless to say, these national marriage markets also drew legions of young men in search of dowries.

Family gatherings, particularly weddings, provided other opportunities to introduce young people to each other. A bachelor's *Tischdame,* the woman seated next to him at dinner, was most often an eligible young lady. Even when these events took place in distant cities, they were considered important enough that if the entire family could not afford to attend, the marriage-aged member would be sent to represent the rest. There were many instances of young couples first meeting at friends' or relatives' weddings.[142]

Even when families no longer had the power to impose partners on their offspring, they often instigated their children's search or introduced "acceptable" young people to each other. As late as 1920, a young Berlin woman who would have married the young man of her choice had he not died, consented to meet a man introduced to her by a family friend. They met "by coincidence" in a restaurant and he visited her at home for about a half year. On their own, they decided to marry. The families were delighted with the "good match" (*gute Partie*): a substantial dowry for a successful professional. The couple really liked each other as well.[143] Such marriages entailed a bit more volition and initiative by the individuals than traditionally arranged marriages. They often involved people who might have met a partner on their own. But, prior to World War I, arranged marriages and cover-ups still predominated.

That is not to say that love relationships did not exist. One can find traces of such marriages even prior to the Imperial period.[144] Still, most spontaneous decisions to marry, particularly those that involved no dowry, can be found only after 1900. Female university students and women involved in youth movements were more prone to choose their own partners and to reject the "tragedy of arranged marriages. . .based on money, income or position."[145] This may be explained partly by the independence it took to enter academia or join the youth movement, either of which implied resistance to traditional parental values or the acceptance of exceptional social behavior by parents; and partly by their meeting more single males. In such cases, companionate marriages based on complementary interests followed. Mutual concerns and activities, rather than traditional considerations of finance, became the basis for marriage.[146] Yet, then, as now, choices almost always fell within parameters set by parental expectations and childhood and adolescent socialization. Also, they sought their parents' blessings.[147] If all social, financial, geographical, health, educational and personality preconditions were met, parents might give their consent even if they did not particularly like their child's selection.[148]

Dowries were not vital to love relationships. In earlier eras, the couple would wait until the groom had saved enough to maintain a family. One such couple who met in 1890 had to wait seven years before the village teacher could support a wife.[149] Another couple had to wait three years until the woman's older sisters had been married. She had fallen in love "out of turn" and could not embarrass her older sisters by preceding them to the altar. In this case, the postponement also allowed the groom to build up his finances.[150] In these partnerships, then, the emphasis was on "love" and the groom's ability to earn, rather than on the bride's wealth. This does not mean, however, that dowries were entirely ignored. In 1912, for example, neighbors in a small town agreed to marry after a seven year courtship. Even though the bride and groom were "in love," their parents initiated financial discussions. The bride's father, a cigar merchant, and the groom's father, a cattle dealer, decided on the woman's dowry, 15,000 M. plus a house. Parents often insisted upon dowries as a contribution to the new household or as an indication of the status of the bride and her family.[151] So even love matches, which ignored the traditional formalities of arrangement and financial inquiry, often included optional, rather than compulsory, dowries.

Urban, working-class Jews were the only Jews who did not formally arrange their marriages, either for property, status or religious reasons. While the lack of substantial property is obvious, religious motivations are more obscure. Compared to the urban middle class, urban workers intermarried more.[152] Most likely, property provided a cudgel to keep middle-class offspring within the familial and communal fold, and the lack of property allowed—or forced—poorer Jews to marry out. Dowries (or the threat of losing them if one intermarried against parents' desires) thus maintained inter-group solidarity. However, intermarriage was not only a function of economics, since poor, rural Jews intermarried less than their urban counterparts. It was also a function of culture and milieu. The more cohesive rural Jewish community and family were also more religious and restrictive. Isolated from many modern challenges—although not from migration—they attempted to guide their young firmly in traditional ways. Urban society, on the other hand, was more open and more secular. It offered its young workers more personal freedom and greater opportunities to meet potential spouses. Peer groups became the focal point of social activity for young working women, whether they lived alone or with their families. Factory jobs, white-collar work in retail shops, government offices, private business and industry presented opportunities unavailable to the cloistered bourgeois *höhere Tochter* or the rural cattle dealer's daughter. Casual meetings at work and at social clubs did lead to liaisons and marriage. Eyeing her working class sisters with some envy, one bourgeois woman (born 1905, Berlin) recalled that she had been taught to "pin down a man. Love is nothing." Yet, "poor people, they fell in love. He worked and she worked. But I was not in that circle. We were brought up to get married."[153] While this is a rose-colored version of working class marriage, it suggests that propertyless marriages allowed women relatively more choice—within the limits set by class and gender—than marriages in which property and status were the primary considerations.[154]

On the spectrum between the extremes of traditionally arranged marriages between utter strangers and those initiated by individual choice lay marriages between relatives, usually cousins (*Verwandtenehen).* Families consolidated and strengthened their bonds through these marriages. Some of these unions were arranged by parents in a traditional manner, others were initiated by the individuals who had known each other for many years, and still others arose as a result of carefully planned family events. Brokers were unnecessary, since each side knew the partners. Often young people had met at family occasions in distant cities, had visited each other's homes for vacations or when traveling or studying and had heard of each other's lives through family correspondence. To meet through family networks was not unusual, since it was typical of Jewish families, even those of very modest means, to send their children on family visits. As marriage age drew near, young people sometimes took advantage of a family gathering to observe each other as potential partners. For some, this opportunity may have been preferable to the impending introduction to a total stranger, although, sometimes the cousins were relative strangers themselves. Still, a sense of familiarity, of shared backgrounds, may have made a marriage decision somewhat easier for both individuals. And, occasionally, the cousins had been old friends. (One couple had known each other so long that the wife remembered her husband helping her with her school essays.)[155]

Jews were the religious denomination most disposed to such relationships. In Prussia, between 1872 and 1875, for example, fourteen per 1000 marriages among Protestants, ten per 1000 among Catholics, and twenty-three per 1000 among Jews were between two relatives.[156] Cousin marriages were a recourse employed, in particular, by small-town Jews with little or no means at their disposal. Without money or wide-ranging social networks, they looked to the family for mates. Their wealthier Jewish neighbors, with wider business and social contacts, resorted to these marriages less frequently.[157] When wealthier cousins did marry, it was generally thought that they were trying "to keep the money in the family."[158] Since Jews were heavily engaged in business and commerce, marital alliances could potentially consolidate businesses and expand markets. Thus, it is likely that dowries were used to preserve family wealth.

Cousin marriages were also a strategem that was frequently unavoidable and often appealing for a minority intent on preserving its religious distinctiveness. Unlike Christians, for whom the marriage pool was substantial, it was occasionally necessary for Jews to marry relatives because other choices were limited. Also, unlike Catholics, who needed special Church dispensation, Jewish society accepted cousin marriages. There were no sanctions by the religion or the culture.[159] Despite genetic dangers, there were potentially more rewards for entering such marriages and greater punishments (i.e., not marrying) for foregoing them than among the non-Jewish population.

The primacy of property in marriage decisions would be successfully challenged only after World War I. Then, the economic, geographic and social mobility and the concomitant increase in personal decision making of a modern market economy, already discernible in the Imperial era but not fully developed until later, contributed to more independent marriage decisions. Furthermore, successive waves of war, inflation and depression hurt the savings of middle class families. Very few daughters had dowries to offer. Finally, and importantly, women's independent earnings and earning potential began to replace dowries. In Imperial Germany, however, traditional patterns persisted. German middle class families pursued economic and social goals as they married off their children. Wealthy Germans arranged property transfers with the marriage of their offspring. The lower middle class struggled to save up for dowries. Only among the poorest were property exchanges and arrangements uncommon.

For Jews, this picture was complicated by religous, regional and class factors. Marriage had symbolic and religious meaning, since marriage was one of the few crucial turning points where one affirmed or rejected one's group affiliation. Thus, Jews exerted great energy in pursuit of endogamy. But marriage was also an opportunity to improve or maintain economic status. Thus, Jewish practices reflected the continued importance of property in the middle class marriage bargain, despite changing ideologies regarding love. As the rhetoric of romance proceeded apace in the early twentieth century, both urban and rural Jews attempted to accommodate to the dominant culture and avoid criticism by covering up arranged marriages. The lengths to which they went in order to make "coincidence" out of preplanned arrangements indicated their recognition of the imbalance between social ideology and Jewish practice. Further, it reflected their desire to mitigate antisemitic accusations and to fit into what they believed to be a general consensus on marriage. However, as much as they may have preferred to adapt to changing social ideology and social norms, their minority status, religious beliefs and economic profile made such adjustments difficult and, often, impossible. In fact, although they adopted some of the language and facade of modern marriage practices, the tenacity of Jewish marriage customs in Imperial Germany suggests the extent to which Jews resisted complete assimilation into German society and the extent to which the Jewish and German bourgeoisies, for very practical reasons, both lagged behind—while often promoting—a romantic version of marriage.

REFERENCES

Research for this essay was supported by a grant from the Deutsche Forschungsgemeinschaft and by a Leo Baeck Institute Research Fellowship. I wish to thank the staffs of the Leo Baeck Institute, New York, and the Central Archives for the History of the Jewish People, Jerusalem, for their help. I am also indebted to the members of the German Women's History Study Group, New York, for their careful reading of an earlier version of this essay. Finally, my appreciation goes to Paula Hyman and Jay Kaplan for their comments and encouragement.

Since the topic of love and marriage is a sensitive one, some people who gave interviews preferred to remain anonymous. I have used an initial, instead of a name, where this was the case.

Abbreviations

ALBI. . . . . .Archives of the Leo Baeck Institute, New York
AZJ. . . . .*Allgemeine Zeitung des Judentums,* Berlin
LBI. . . . . .Leo Baeck Institute, library, New York
ZDSJ. . . . .*Zeitschrift für Demographie und Statistik der Juden,* Berlin

REFERENCE NOTES

1. Lawrence Schofer, ''Emancipation and Population Change,'' in Werner E. Mosse, Arnold Paucker, et. al., *Revolution and Evolution: 1848 in German-Jewish History* (Tübingen, 1981), 83.

2. Despite the notorious, but relatively few, marriages between wealthy Jewish women and impecunious nobles, we can assume that most intermarriages were *not* arranged by Jewish parents. Conversely, the low rate of intermarriage points to the likelihood of careful arrangements. As late as 1916, when commenting upon the small number of Jewish women involved in mixed marriges, Jewish demographers suggested the reason for this was the ''usual way of getting married among the Jews, namely arranged marriages.'' *Zeitschrift für Demographie und Statistik der Juden* (hereafter *ZDSJ*), 12 (April/June 1916): 56.

3. Elise Polko, *Unsere Pilgerfahrt von der Kinderstube bis zum eigenen Herd* (Leipzig, 1863), 128, 133.

4. Ann Taylor Allen, ''Sex and Satire in Wilhelmine Germany: *'Simplicissimus'* Looks at Family Life,'' *Journal of European Studies* 7 (1977): 29.

5. This was not only the case in Germany. See, Bonnie Smith, *Ladies of the Leisure Class: The Bourgeoises of Northern France in the Nineteenth Century* (Princeton, 1981), 57. See also Erna Hellerstein, Leslie Parker, et. al. eds., *Victorian Women: A Documentary Account of Women's Lives in Nineteenth-Century England, France, and the United States* (Stanford, 1981), 140-142.

6. Sometimes the terms *Mitgift, Aussteuer* or *Ausstattung* were used interchangeably. It is necessary to examine the context of the statement in which they appear to see if they mean wealth and property or linen and furniture.

7. David Sabean, ''Verwandtschaft und Familie in einem württembergischen Dorf 1500 bis 1870: einige methodische Überlegungen,'' in Werner Conze (ed.), *Sozialgeschichte der Familie in der Neuzeit Europas* (Stuttgart, 1976), 244. A surplus of embroidered linens was a sign of both wealth and diligence: an indication of the bride's leisure time and of her industriousness.

8. Jewish families invited neighbors in as well. One woman recalled the display of her sixty-four hand-embroidered pillow cases along with embroidered sheets, blanket covers, towels and handkerchiefs. Interviews with A. Hamburger (born 1888, Württemberg), New Jersey, June 1981, March 1982. The custom of displaying the trousseau seems common in other societies too. See, for example, Jane Lambiri-Dimaki essay and Jane Schneider essay in this volume.

9. Toni Ehrlich, unpublished memoirs, Leo Baeck Institute, New York (hereafter LBI), no. 85, p. 62.

10. Describing a middle-class trousseau of the 1890s, Toni Ehrlich recalled dozens of bedroom linens, tablecloths and household linens. The latter included special towels for dishes, glasses, knives, silver, bathrooms, windows and combs. *Ibid.* As late as World War I, women took great pride in their embroidered linens, but already by the 1890s some purchased their trousseaux from stores. Clara Sander recorded that her sister's trousseau (Frankfurt/Main, 1892) was store-bought and that her mother's had been entirely handmade twenty-five years earlier. Clara Sander, unpublished memoirs, LBI, no. 344, p. 64.

11. To understand the cost of a 2,000 to 3,000 M. trousseau it is useful to know that a family of six could spend about 2,400 to 3,100 M. a year on food between 1900 and 1905. Margarete Freudenthal, *Gestaltwandel der städtischen, bürgerlichen und proletarischen Hauswirtschaft unter besonderer Berücksichtigung des Typenwandels von Frau und Familie* (Würzburg, 1934) 140. For a complete description of a *standesgemäss* (class appropriate) trousseau, see the list from *Das Blatt gehört der Hausfrau* (1901) in Ingeborg Weber-Kellermann, *Die deutsche Familie: Versuch einer Sozialgeschichte* (Frankfurt/Main, 1974), 113-14.

12. Wilhelm Riehl, *Die Familie,* vol. 3 *Die Naturgeschichte des Volkes als Grundlage einer deutschen Social-Politik,* 9th ed. (Stuttgart, 1882), 180.

13. Schofer, ''Emancipation and Population Change,'' 83.

14. Some of these exceptions included the marriages of the Berlin salon women in the late eighteenth century.

15. *The Memoirs of Glückel of Hameln,* trans. Marvin Lowenthal (New York, 1977), 96 (from the Talmud, *Sota,* 2-a).

16. By 1794, the *Allgemeine Preussische Landrecht* codified what may already have become common behavior: parents could not force children to marry a particular partner, and both parties had to give their free consent. Ute Gerhard, *Verhältnisse und Verhinderungen. Frauenarbeit, Familie und Rechte der Frauen im 19. Jahrhundert* (Frankfurt/Main, 1978), 86. As of 1875, the Prussian law allowed women over the age of twenty-four to marry without parental permission. The German Civil Code of 1896 eliminated penalties for a broken engagement. Before this, laws had made engagements binding and a betrothal was taken as seriously as a marriage ceremony. Jewish custom had also viewed the betrothal as binding. See: Jacob Katz, "Family, Kinship, and Marriage among Ashkenazim in the sixteenth to eighteenth Centuries," *Jewish Journal of Sociology* 1 (1959): 5-6.

17. Rahel Straus, *Wir Lebten in Deutschland: Erinnerungen einer deutschen Jüdin, 1880-1933* (Stuttgart, 1962), 104.

18. Lucy Maas, unpublished memoirs, LBI, 8, 10, 18.

19. Flora Goldschmidt, unpublished memoirs, LBI, p. 17. The family lived in Breslau.

20. Jacob Rosenheim, *Erinnerungen 1870-1920,* ed. Heinrich Eisenmann and Herbert N. Kruskal (Frankfurt/Main, 1970), 66-67.

21. Straus, *Wir Lebten in Deutschland,* 104.

22. Clara Geismar, unpublished memoirs, LBI, #126, p. 112.

23. Charlotte Hamburger-Liepmann, "Geschichte der Familien Liepmann und Bleichroeder," unpublished memoirs, LBI, n. p.

24. Josef Lange, unpublished memoir, LBI, p. 44.

25. See, for examples: *General Anzeiger für die gesamten Interessen des Judentums* (Berlin), March 19, 1903, supplement, or *Handwerk und Gewerbe* (Berlin), June 1915, back cover.

26. Simon Bischheim, unpublished memoir, LBI no. 42, p. 4. The author was born in Frankfurt/Main in 1886.

27. Alice Goldstein, "Some Demographic Characteristics of Village Jews in Germany: Nonnenweier, 1800-1931," in Paul Ritterband, ed., *Modern Jewish Fertility,* vol. 1 *Studies in Judaism in Modern Times,* ed. Jacob Neusner (Leiden, 1981). This may have been a more general pattern. A study of Greece also suggests that brothers often went so far as to give their sisters part of their inheritance in order to enable them to marry. It was, of course, in the brother's interest to find a prestigious match for his sister. Ernestine Friedl, *Vasilika, a Village in Modern Greece* (New York, 1962).

28. Isidor Hirschfeld memoirs, in Monika Richarz, ed. *Jüdisches Leben in Deutschland. Selbstzeugnisse zur Sozialgeschichte im Kaiserreich* (Stuttgart, 1979). 248-49.

29. Hermann Schwab, *Jewish Rural Communities in Germany* (London, 1956), 15.

30. Perles collection, ALBI, #ARB, 414, 4884, 25, 38-39. I would like to thank Ismar Schorsch for calling my attention to this collection.

31. Herman Pollack, *Jewish Folkways in Germanic Lands (1648-1806)* (Cambridge, Mass., 1971), 31.

32. Gustav Jacoby collection, ALBI, #ARC 1120, 2943.

33. Ads such as "Broker, well-known in better circles. . ." can be found in: *Israelitisches Gemeindeblatt,* Oct. 27, 1905, ad page; *Das jüdische Blatt* (Ansbach/Strassburg), 16; or *General Anzeiger,* Jan. 25, 1904, ad page.

34. *Handwerk und Gewerbe,* Jan. 1915, p. 129, *Israelitisches Gemeindeblatt,* Oct. 13, 1905, p. 409. For a detective's report, see: Pinkus collection, ALBI, #AR7030, box 5, folder 7, a letter dated June 20, 1910.

35. Richarz, *Jüdisches Leben in Deutschland,* 2:21.

36. Utz Jeggle, *Judendörfer in Württemberg* (Tübingen, 1969), 281.

37. Salomon Andorn, unpublished memoir, LBI, no. 414, p. 13. Andorn writes of the 1870s. He lived in a village of 1,200 people in Hesse.

38. William Wertheimer, *Zwischen zwei Welten, Der Förster von Brooklyn (Lebenserinnerungen des ehemaligen jüdischen Lehrers in. . .Baden)* (Passau, 1966), 24. See also, Andorn memoir, LBI no. 413, 4-5.

39. Andorn, no. 414, p. 13-14. This was the case among Eastern European Jews as well. In their study of the shtetl, researchers note that brokers were the butt of many jokes. Mark Zborowski and Elizabeth Herzog, *Life is With People: The Culture of the Shtetl* (New York, 1952). 271-73.

40. *Frankfurter Israelitisches Familienblatt,* Oct. 18, 1907, p. 13.

41. Fabius Schach, in *Israelitisches Wochenblatt* (Berlin), Jan. 19, 1912, p. 2.

42. *General Anzeiger,* June 27, 1904, advertisement page. Although these samples run only as high as 100,000 M., there were advertisements in non-Jewish papers, such as the *Frankfurter Zeitung und Handelsblatt,* in which Jews also advertised, that ran as high as 300,000 M. See, for example, papers from July 1914. For purposes of comparison, it should be noted that in 1904 a higher civil servant (*Justizbeamter*) could earn about 8,700 M. a year. Freudenthal, *Gestaltwandel,* 132.

43. *General Anzeiger,* March 21, 1904, supplement. It was not uncommon for more to be promised "at a later date." Fathers promised money at the marriage and then after their deaths as part of the inheritance. See, for example, Graetz letter to Perles, 1884, regarding his daughter-in-law's marriage settlement: 200,000 M. at the wedding and 300,000 M. upon her father's death. Perles collection ALBI, no. ARB 414, 4884. Also, among the very wealthy, were those who gave a generous sum and then yearly stipends. See: Ehevertrag, Hans Sachs collection, ALBI, no. ARC907, 2566, II/25 (1880).

44. Interview with Mrs. X (born *circa* 1900, Berlin), New York, June 1981.

45. Interview with Mrs—(born 1905, Berlin) in John Foster, *Community of Fate: German-Jews in Melbourne,* forthcoming. The idea of marrying for a good home was certainly not unique to Jews, but was a matter of course for most European bourgeois families. The grandmother's advice was remarkably similar to that given by the *Family Herald* (London, 1856) to a governess who had received a proposal from a man forty years her senior. The *Herald* suggested, "It is merely a question of expediency, as marriage in general is: it is 'Can I do better—would it be better to accept a home of this kind than to run the risk of having none at all?' Women all reason thus, and so do men. The ideal of love is never realised. . .if it is, danger awaits it, for perfect satisfaction is of short duration on this planet." Sally Mitchell, "The Forgotten Woman of the Period," in Martha Vicinus, ed., *A Widening Sphere: Changing Roles of Victorian Women* (Bloomington, 1977),

46. *General Anzeiger,* May 30, 1904.

47. Ibid.

48. Freudenthal, *Gestaltwandel,* 138-39; *General Anzeiger,* Jan. 29, 1903, p. 4.

49. *General Anzeiger,* May 30, 1904.

50. For example, a craftsman might accept 7,000 M. with a woman who was also "enterprising." *General Anzeiger,* June 20, 1904; Jan. 29, 1903, p. 4; March 19, 1903, supplement.

51. *General Anzeiger,* March 21, 1904, supplement.

52. *General Anzeiger,* Jan. 13, 1907.

53. See: Felix A. Theilhaber, *Die Schädigung der Rasse durch soziales und wirtschaftliches Aufsteigen bewiesen an den Berliner Juden* (Berlin: 1914), 87-88; *ZDSJ* (February-March 1915): 52-54. Among Jews, the very richest and the very poorest intermarried relatively more than those in the middle. Among the richest, families paid dearly in order to enter Gentile high society. For the poorest women, intermarriage may have been the only option, since Jewish men, in short supply, preferred women with dowries. It would be worth investigation to see if the decline of dowries was related to an increase in intermarriage.

54. Adolf Riesenfeld collection, ALBI, diary p. 98. We should distinguish the groom's "worth," that is, *his* money or value in job or property from "brideprice." The latter was an economic exchange tendered to the woman's family. In both cases the man had to show something of value, but in industrial societies *he* kept it and promised only to maintain his wife.

55. *Frankfurter Israelitisches Gemeindeblatt,* October 18, 1907, pp. 3 13.

56. *General Anzeiger,* Jan. 15, 1903, supplement.

57. *Das jüdische Blatt,* Feb. 28, 1914, p. 14.

58. Schwab, *Jewish Rural Communities,* 82. Interview with A. Hamburger, married in 1912.

59. *Das jüdische Blatt,* June 26, 1915, and *Israelitsche Gemeindeblatt,* Oct. 13, 1905, p. 409, respectively.

60. *General Anzeiger,* December 4, 1902, supplement.

61. The examples and conclusion were offered by Bruno Stern, interview, New York, 1980 (born in 1912, Niederstettin, Württemberg).

62. Jeggle, *Judendörfer in Württemberg,* 281. In this same period, the migration of Gentile women was linked to marriage or to the demand for domestic servants, whereas men migrated in response to modern labor market conditions. John Knodel and Mary Jo Maynes, "Urban and Rural Marriage Patterns in Imperial Germany," in *Journal of Family History* 1 (1976): 144.

63. Theilhaber, *Die Schädigung,* 88-89. Jack Goody has suggested that the later marriage age of European women may have been connected to the necessity of accumulating dowries. Jack Goody and S.J. Tambiah, *Bridewealth and Dowry* (Cambridge 1973), 10. In explaining the late age at marriage of Jews, demographers have usually pointed to men's need to establish businesses or careers. It is also likely that dowries delayed marriage.

64. Choices for spinsters were very limited. Until the turn of the century, women had no education which would have enabled them to earn their own living. As late as 1907, there were only 150,000 white collar jobs available to middle-class women. (Werner Conze, "Sozialgeschichte 1850-1918," in Hermann Aubin and Wolfgang Zorn, eds., *Handbuch der deutschen Wirtschafts und Sozialgeschichte* (Stuttgart, 1976), 635. Thus, many ended up as governesses. A Jewish woman wrote that the tragedy of her friends' lives "was that their father went bankrupt. Both girls had to take care of themselves and because they had not been trained to do anything, the only class-appropriate job they could consider was that of governess; their marriage chances were minimal because there was no dowry." (Elberfeld, 1890's, in Hamburger-Liepmann, "Geschichte der Familien," 74.) Those who could not support themselves frequently lived with their parents, and, later, with their brother's or sister's family. This was the case among other Germans too: "in 'good bourgeois families' there were hordes of girls who remained unmarried. . .tied to the households of parents or brothers. . ." (Rolf Engelsing, *Zur Sozialgeschichte deutscher Mittel-und Unterschichten* (Göttingen, 1973), 41.) Decrying the position of "old maids" the heroine of a feminist novel painted the following portrait as she argued in favor of careers for women: ". . .it must be horrible to be an old maid, whose. . .life is nothing but a demoralizing parasitism. First the parents have to feed the reject much longer than they wish; then the brother or brother-in-law plays the role of the provider; then the relatives, and, if they don't own anything or if there aren't any relatives, the community. . .has to. . .care. . . .Fortunately one does not yet let them die on the street; that is worth a lot. . ." (in Aimeé Duc, *Sind es Frauen?* (Berlin, 1903), trans. by Lillian Faderman and Brigitte Eriksson, *Lesbian-Feminism in Turn-of-the-Century Germany* (Tallahassee, Fla., 1980), 11.

65. See: Steven Lowenstein, "Results of Atlas Investigations among Jews of Germany," in Marvin Herzog, et al. eds., *The Field of Yiddish: Studies in Language, Folklore and Literature* 3 (London, 1969), 24. Also, memoirs and interviews point this out.

66. This was the case among propertied peasants as well. See Sabean, "Verwandtschaft und Familie, 242.

67. Interview with A. Hamburger.

68. *Brockhaus: Conversations-Lexikon,* 13th ed., (1885), 11: 771, and 14th ed. (1902), 11: 935.

69. Conrad Rosenstein, unpublished memoirs, LBI, no. 328, p. 12. He was born in Berlin in 1910.

70. Karl Ettlinger, *Moritzchens Tagebuch* (Berlin, 1908), 138-39. The events took place in the first decade of the twentieth century.

71. See, for example: Ehevertrag, Elkan Family collection, ALBI, no. ARC 700/1960, no. 17. Contract from 1867. Collection includes the official receipts for the dowry and the trousseau signed by the groom.

72. See: Ehevertrag, Sinn Family collection, ALBI , no. ARC406/1163, IV, no. 1. Contract from 1867.

73. See: Elkan Family collection and Walter Harold collection, ALBI, no. ARC 4156, II, no. 20. Contract from 1872. I would like to thank Erika Grossmann for helping me translate these documents.

74. For example, in 1884 one man hoped to avert his daughter-in-law's (and son's) disinheritance by asking the original witness to testify to her father's spoken promise. By this time, then, spoken promises may have begun to replace written contracts with the understanding that the spoken word was as binding as the written one. Perles collection, 7172.

75. Hirschfeld, in Richarz, *Jüdisches Leben in Deutschland,* 2: 249.

76. Marie Maas, unpublished memoirs, LBI #257, 40-48. She was born in Breslau in 1855. At the turn of the century, a highly placed civil servant paid 300 M. a year for this insurance. Freudenthal, *Gestaltwandel,* 137.

77. Geismar, memoirs, 97. In 18th century Hamburg, the Jewish community insisted that relatives help the needy. Pollack, *Jewish Folkways in Germanic Lands,* 32.

78. Diane Owen Hughes, "From Brideprice to Dowry in Mediterranean Europe," in this volume.

79. Pollack, *Jewish Folkways in Germanic Lands,* 32.

80. Jacobson collection, ALBI, II, no.42.

81. Hamburg and Altona: Hamburg Staatsarchiv, "Jüdische Gemeinde," 522-1, Ehesachen; Würzburg: records of the Feist Hirsch Berg'schen Aussteuer Stiftung, Central Archives for the History of the Jewish People, Jerusalem, Rep. WR, nos. 909-972; Lübeck: Central Archives, GA II/541. These clubs were also found in smaller towns and villages.

82. For example, the Verein zur Ausstattung jüdischer Bräute (Cologne) agreed to give a 3,000 M. dowry to brides nominated by its members. This club had a membership of 130 people, annual dues of 1,103 M., and fixed assets. Other clubs gave less. *Israelitisches Gemeindeblatt,* March 1, 1912, 92.

83. Wertheimer, *Zwischen zwei Welten,* 25.

84. Rosenstein memoir, p. 2. This was in Berlin in 1870. Unless they were wealthy, widows with children did not remarry as easily as widowers. The latter could choose from a pool of widows as well as young marriage-aged women. For orphanage, see: Staatsarchiv Königsberg, Rep. 2, II, #3, 194, p. 59, Geheimes Staatsarchiv Preussischer Kulturbesitz, Berlin.

85. Riesenfeld collection, diary entry of May 11, 1916 referring to Breslau in the 1890s.

86. *Israelitisches Gemeindeblatt,* June 24, 1892, pp. 204-7.

87. Geismar, memoirs, 112. She was referring to the 1860s and 1870s.

88. Liselotte Stern, in Monika Richarz, ed., *Jüdisches Leben in Deutschland, Selbstzeugnisse zur Sozialgeschichte, 1919-1945* (Stuttgart: 1982), 168-171.

89. In order to discover if Jewish women were, in fact, being "left behind," we would have to examine population, intermarriage and conversion statistics and marriage frequency. Where possible, it would then be useful to compare these to those of the general population. At the turn of the century, Germany, like most West European countries, had a population in which there were more women than men. In 1900, there were 1,033 women to 1,000 men. As for intermarriage, Jewish men led the way. (*ZDSJ,* March 1913, p. 44). The percentage of Jewish grooms contracting mixed marriages in Prussia grew from 4 percent in 1875-79 to 8 percent in 1895-99, to 24 percent in 1915-19, leaving fewer available Jewish husbands. (This data was computed from the official statistics and communicated to me by Professor U. O. Schmelz, Institute of Contemporary Jewry, The Hebrew University of Jerusalem). Among converts, men—particularly during marrying years (20 to 40)—again took the lead. (*ZDSJ,* June 1909, pp. 88-89). Thus, population statistics alone would seem to substantiate these worries. If one then examines the frequency of Jewish marriages, preliminary conclu-

sions (which need further investigation) also indicate that Jewish women were being "left behind." For example, in 1903, fewer Jews married relative to their population than non-Jews. Only 70 per 10,000 Jews (including those in intermarriages) married compared to 82 per 10,000 Christians. (*ZDSJ*, April 1905, p. 8). In 1906, 82 per 10,000 Christians and 74 per 10,000 Jews married. Since Jews had a relatively greater marriage-aged population than non-Jews, the Jewish population married even less frequently than these percentages indicate. (*ZDSJ*, December 1908, p. 189). It remains the task of future investigators to discover the number of Jewish and Gentile women remaining single at given ages throughout the Imperial era before we can substantiate these observations. For the year 1880, we can find the singulate mean age at marriage for men and women in Germany and measures of German nuptuality in John Knodel and Mary Jo Maynes, "Marriage Patterns," 162-68.

90. *Allgemeine Zeitung des Judentums* (hereafter AZJ), 1849, pp. 203-205.

91. *Die Laubhütte* (Regensburg), July 18, 1895, p. 336.

92. *Israelitisches Familienblatt*, July 31, 1919, p. 10.

93. Sidonie Werner in *Im deutschen Reich*, February 1914, pp. 53-54.

94. This theme was already a cliché in the Greek comedies of 300 B.C. *Gedichte und Scherze in jüdischer Mundart*, Bloch Publishers, Berlin, n.d., pamphlet nos. 18, 23.

95. Ibid., pamphlet no. 7, pp. 8-10.

96. Georg Hermann, *Henriette Jacoby* (Berlin 1915), 22.

97. Ettlinger, *Moritzchen*, 123-24.

98. Artur Landsberger, *Millionäre* (Berlin 1913), 326-27.

99. On Gentile criticism of the Jewish "dowry chase" see, also: Henry Wassermann, "The Fliegende Blätter as a Source for the Social History of German Jewry," *Yearbook of the Leo Baeck Institute*, 1983, 123-24.

100. Adolph Asch in Richarz, Jüdisches Leben in Deutschland 2: 224.

101. Jeggle, *Judendörfer in Württemberg*, 165.

102. *Simplicissimus*, 2 (1897-1898). 36: 284-85; 5 (1900-01). 9:69 and 47: 377.

103. Alice Berend, *Die Gute Alte Zeit:Bürger and Spiessbürger im 19. Jahrhundert* (Hamburg, 1962), 66.

104. *Frankfurter Zeitung und Handelsblatt*, July 26, 1914, p. 3; July 30, 1914, p. 5; August 2, 1914, p. 3.

105. Ibid., August 2, 1914, p. 3.

106. *Allgemeine Zeitung München*, April 18, 1885, p. 1576.

107. *Frankfurter Zeitung und Handelsblatt*, July 26, 1914, pp. 7, 12. *Berliner Illustriere Zeitung*, January 18, 1914, p. 41.

108. *Frankfurter Zeitung und Handelsblatt*, August 2, 1914, p. 3.

109. Berthold Auerbach, *Barfüssele* (Berlin 1912).

110. Wilhelm Riehl, *Die Familie*, vol. 3 *Die Naturgeschichte*, 13.

111. Robert Lee, "Family and 'Modernisation': The Peasant Family and Social Change in Nineteenth-Century Bavaria," in Richard Evans and W. R. Lee, eds., *The German Family* (London, 1981), 95.

112. Gerhard Wilke and Kurt Wagner, "Family and Household: Social Structures in a German Village between the Two World Wars," in Evans and Lee, *The German Family*, 137. Most likely, the matchmakers in question were Jews. Jews were heavily involved in the rural economy as cattle dealers, and Jeggle's findings for Württemberg, that Jews brokered Christian marriages, probably holds for other rural areas as well.

113. Johanna Harris, in Richarz, *Jüdisches Leben in Deutschland* 2:162.

114. Wilke and Wagner, "Family and Household," 139.

115. Jeggle, *Judendörfer in Württemberg*, 220, 225-26.

116. This continued well into the 1920s in some of the smallest towns. Interview with L. Stern (born 1922, Weikersheim, Württemberg), New York, December 1982.

117. Henry Mayhew, *German Life and Manners as Seen in Saxony at the Present Day* (London, 1865), quoted in Priscilla Robertson, *An Experience of Women: Pattern and Change in Nineteenth Century Europe* (Philadelphia, 1982), 81.

118. Karen Horney, *The Adolescent Diaries of Karen Horney* (New York, 1980), 61-62.

119. *Akademisch gebildete Beamten* ranged from *Referendar* to *Oberpräsidenten.* Hansjoachim Henning, *Das westdeutsche Bürgertum in der Epoche der Hochindustrialisierung, 1860-1914: Soziales Verhalten und Soziale Strukturen,* Teil I: *Das Bildungsbürgertum in den Preussischen Westprovinzen* (Wiesbaden, 1972), 294, 331, 383.

120. Ibid., 274, and Karin Hausen, "Die Polarisierung der 'Geschlechtscharaktere'—Eine Spiegelung der Dissoziation von Erwerbs-und Familienleben," in Conze, *Sozialgeschichte,* 384.

121. Henning, *Das westdeutsche Bürgertum,* 432, 460-61.

122. Ibid., 393, 454, 460. The desire to save for substantial future dowries may have been another cause for the decline in Jewish fertility in this period.

123. Claudia Hahn, "Der öffentliche Dienst und die Frauen-Beamtinnen in der Weimarer Republik," in Frauengruppe Faschismusforschung, eds., *Mutterkreuz und Arbeitsbuch: Zur Geschichte der Frauen in der Weimarer Republik und im Nationalsozialismus* (Frankfurt/Main, 1981), 51.

124. After World War I, dowries and the arrangements that went with them became much less common in Germany. Jews, in contrast to non-Jews, may have clung longer to arranged marriages in order to assure endogamy in a small pool of available partners. Also, as a result of their heavy participation in business and commerce, many Jews continued to demand dowries throughout the 1920s. In the 1920s Ruppin remarked that the dowry was much less common among Christians than among Jews. (Arthur Ruppin, *Soziologie der Juden* (Berlin, 1930), 221). This does not, however, imply that love matches ignored financial issues. In 1952, 65 percent of a sample of German women claimed to have brought a dowry into their marriages. William J. Goode, *World Revolution and Family Patterns* (New York, 1970), 34.

125. Hughes, "From Brideprice to Dowry," in this volume.

126. Fritz Stern, *Gold and Iron: Bismarck, Bleichröder, and the Building of the German Empire* (New York, 1977), 462.

127. Henning, *Das westdeutsche Bürgertum,* 334.

128. Max Weber quoted by Stern, *Gold and Iron,* 468.

129. This does not mean that Jews were unaware of upward social mobility within their *own* community. However, Jewish and non-Jewish *perceptions* differed here: outsiders were unlikely to recognize marriage to another Jew, no matter what her or his family's position, as an increase in *social* status, since it was not a marriage into the "German" elite.

130. See for example, Riehl *(Die Familie,* 46) who was prescribing, rather than describing, when he said that love marriages were the rule in his time. (This book was published first in 1858, 9th ed. published in 1882.)

131. Jacob Katz, paper delivered at the National Jewish Family Center of the American Jewish Committee, March 18, 1982.

132. Riesenfeld collection, ALBI. He became engaged around 1907 in Breslau. Unfortunately, memoirs give a rather one-sided, positive view of the engagement period. Intended for the children and grandchildren of the author, they rarely disclose the fears, anxieties or anger that might have accompanied such marriage transactions and engagement rituals.

133. This pretense of spontaneity was sometimes followed by a pretense of ignorance regarding financial matters. Marianne Weber (born 1870) recalled that dowries were important, but girls were not supposed to know about them. Robertson, *Experience of Women,* 81. Some, in fact, did not. Others knew, but pretended not to, and many, as we have seen, knew and told of their "worth."

134. Jacob Epstein, unpublished memoirs, LBI, no. 92, p. 31. This took place in Frankfurt/Main in 1881.

135. Riesenfeld collection, Book II, 134-35.

136. Bruno Stern, *Meine Jugenderinnerungen an eine württembergische Kleinstadt und ihre jüdische Gemeinde* (Stuttgart: 1968), 122. He described the period up to 1933.

137. Louis Böhm, *Lieder eines fahrenden Chossid: Humoristische Dichtungen für jüdische Geselligkeit* (Frankfurt/Main, 1922), 17-18.

138. Adolph Asch in Richarz, *Jüdisches Leben in Deutschland,* 2: 227.

139. According to William Goode, since love is potentially disruptive of lineages and class strata, it must be controlled before it appears. There are several patterns by which parents achieve this: child marriage, social segregation of adolescents, formal and informal parental initiatives. The formal pattern permits love to emerge and the informal pattern actually encourages it to. "The Theoretical Importance of Love," in *American Sociological Review* 24 (1959): 38-46.

140. Straus, *Wir Lebten in Deutschland,* 101.

141. By the mid-eighteenth century, major watering places, like Bath, had become marriage markets for a wealthy clientele. By the mid-nineteenth century, Theodore Zeldin described "hordes of mothers and daughters in search of husbands" descending on Vichy. See: Lawrence Stone, *The Family, Sex and Marriage in England, 1500-1800* (New York, 1979), 213 and Zeldin, *France, 1848-1945,* 2 (Oxford, 1977), 93. Max Brod describes the situation of Jewish women on spa "vacations" in *Jüdinnen* (Berlin, 1911).

142. Toni Cassirer, unpublished memoirs, LBI, pp. 12-13. See also Max Gruenewald collection, ALBI, his father's memoirs, which describe how he met his wife at a family wedding in 1890.

143. Interview with Mrs. X.

144. Edmund Hadra, unpublished memoirs, LBI, 88. In previous generations, love relationships occurred infrequently. When they did, parents who consented to the union would employ a matchmaker after the fact "for appearance' sake." Customary negotiations took place, and betrothal documents were signed by both sets of parents. If a young couple fell in love against their parents' wishes, rabbis usually ruled in favor of the parents. Katz, "Family, Kinship and Marriage," 9-10. (For the late eighteenth and the nineteenth centuries, I am purposely excluding the love relationships of untraditional women, such as the participants in the Berlin salons or early feminists.)

I do not mean to imply that there were no love relationships between husbands and wives *after* they married. This can be documented from at least the tenth century through the nineteenth. See, for example, S. D. Goitein, *A Mediterranean Society: the Jewish communities of the Arab world as portrayed in the documents of the Cairo Geniza* (Berkeley, 1978) 3: 165.

145. Straus, *Wir Lebten in Deutschland,* 129. The author attended the University of Heidelberg and married in 1905.

146. Ibid. See also, Charlotte Landau-Muehsam, unpublished memoirs, LBI. She married in Lübeck in 1908.

147. Anna Kronthal, *Posner Mürbekuchen: Jugend Erinnerungen einer Posnerin* (Munich, 1932), 90-93 and Mrs. ——, in Foster, *Community of Fate.*

148. Hadra, memoirs, 200. This took place in Berlin around 1900.

149. Gruenewald collection, ALBI. This took place in a small town in Westphalia.

150. Bertha Katz, unpublished memoirs, LBI, p. 8. Also, Mrs. ——, in Foster, *Community of Fate.* More than sisterly solicitude, the cases of women marrying in birth order indicate the extent of parental control and social convention even when there were no dowries.

151. Interview with A. Hamburger.

152. Theilhaber, *Die Schädigung der Rasse.*

153. Mrs. ——, in Foster, *Community of Fate.* Born in 1905, Berlin.

154. This does not mean that workers had no trousseaus. See, for example, Heilwig Schomerus, "The Family Life-Cycle: A Study of Factory Workers in Nineteenth-Century Württemberg," in Evans, *The German Family.* It remains to be seen whether working class Jewish women brought some savings into marriage. They did marry at a later age (25 to 26 for those marrying craftsmen and 26 for those marrying workers) than their propertied sisters and may have been saving up for marriage. Theilhaber, *Die Schädigung der Rasse.*

155. Sander, memoirs, 62 (born in Frankfurt, married around 1894); Landau-Muehsam memoirs, referring to her sister, married in Lübeck in 1896; Henriette Hirsch in Richarz, *Jüdisches Leben in Deutschland,* 2: 79-80 (met in Halberstadt, married around 1880.)

156. Ruppin, *Soziologie der Juden,* 201; *ZDSJ,* March/April 1924, p. 53. In Hungary and in Alsace-Lorraine, Ruppin showed that Jews married relatives twice as much as non-Jews (pp. 200-201). According to Katz, Jews prohibited marriage only within the innermost

circle of relatives, such as between sister and brother or aunt and nephew (not uncle and niece). "Family, Kinship and Marriage," 14. See also, Goitein, *Mediterranean Society.*

157. Wilhelm Reutlinger, Über die Häufigkeit der Verwandtenehen bei den Juden in Hohenzollern und über Untersuchungen bei Deszendenten aus jüdischen Verwandtenehen," in *Archiv für Rassen-und Gesellschaftsbiologie,* 14 (1922): 303.

158. L. Stern, interview, New York, March 1982.

159. The theme of *Verwandtenehe* appeared frequently in Jewish novels and magazines. It also appeared in non-Jewish literature, e.g., Gabrielle Reuter, *Aus Guter Familie,* 17th. ed., (Berlin, 1908).

Dowry in Modern Greece: An Institution at the Crossroads Between Persistence and Decline

Jane Lambiri-Dimaki

INTRODUCTION

In reviewing current sociological literature on family and marriage, the position of women, and related themes, one cannot help wondering why so little attention has been paid to the institution of the dowry, an institution which still is, after all, part of the social web of a good number of contemporary societies (Ireland, southern Italy, Spain, Portugal, Malta, Greece, Tunisia, Lebanon, etc.).[1]

This neglect is very probably due to the fact that in those countries where sociology and related disciplines are most developed, the institution of the dowry is either altogether unknown (as, for example, in the United States) or has only a limited historical interest, as, for example, in England, Germany, Belgium, and France (where, although it has not been legally abolished, *de facto* French people tend on the whole to regulate property relations between husband and wife on the basis of another legal institution, that of the *communauté de biens).* On the other hand it is in precisely those countries where the institution of the dowry is still alive with manifold economic and social consequences, and where it could become the object of detailed research, that the study of the native social institutions is not favored, because of the underdevelopment of the social sciences.

The purpose of this article is in some small way to help fill this gap in our knowledge of the function and structure of the institution of the dowry in contemporary societies even if only in small part and for only the Greek society.

The material for this study has been drawn mainly from three sources: Greek legal sources (mainly the Greek Civil Code of 1946); the relatively few studies carried out, mainly by American and English social anthropologists, on Greek village life; and personal observation and research data collected in the course of two sociological projects I conducted, one on a Greek provincial town and the other on university students.

STRUCTURE, FUNCTION, AND EFFECTS OF THE INSTITUTION OF THE DOWRY IN MODERN GREECE

The Legal Rules

The dowry is primarily a legal institution, and therefore the examination of its modern structure must take as its starting point the legal rules which govern it. These are contained in the Greek Civil Code, which has applied in this country since 1946.[2] The Greek Civil Code includes a special chapter on dowry (articles 1406-1437); a number of additional articles referring to the dowry are found mainly in the chapters dealing with the relations between parents and children and the rights to inheritance.

The legal definition of the dowry. The following definition of the dowry is given in the Greek Civil Code (article 1406): "Dowry is the property which the wife or somebody else on her behalf gives to the husband in order to alleviate the burdens of marriage." In this definition the main purpose of the dowry is very clearly stated. We note that the modern legislator considers, as has been the case throughout the centuries in this country, that the main function of the dowry is to provide a contribution on the part of the woman to the expenses of marital life.

The rights of the husband and of the wife over the dowry. According to article 1412, the husband, unless stated otherwise in the marriage contract (which is always drawn up before a notary), acquires the right of owning the movable dower property and the right of managing and enjoying the use and advantages (i.e., the usufruct) of the real estate which is part of the dower property. According to article 1414, in case the wife (or whoever acts on her behalf) does not transmit to the husband the right of ownership of the dower property, then he is entitled, as long as the marriage lasts, only to the management and the usufruct of the dower property, while the wife is its real legal owner.

According to articles 1416-1417, the husband is not entitled to alienate either the movable or the real dower property without his wife's consent; when the marriage is dissolved by divorce, the dower property is returned to the wife (or to her heirs), the husband having no more rights over its management (article 1426). In view of these restrictions, it is only too obvious that the dowry is not a gift to the husband.

The obligations of parents vis-à-vis their daughter's endowment. According to article 1495, the father is "obliged to provide his daughter who is about to get married with a dowry proportionate to his wealth, to the number of his children, to his social position, as well as to the social position of the future husband." He can be exempted from this obligation only if it can be proved that by giving a dowry he will become impoverished or that the daughter has some other source of revenue which can provide her with a dowry. In case the father has died or is incapable of providing his daughter with a dowry, this obligation is transferred to the mother (article 1497). Parents have the right to refuse to fulfill this obligation in case their daughter has married without their consent or there are valid reasons for disinheriting her.

It should be noted that the dower property is not given to the daughter as a gift: what is given to her (and through her to her husband) is in fact a part or the whole of what she is legally entitled to inherit one day from her parents. Dowry-giving is indeed a transference of property from the girl's family of origin to her and to her husband, by another means than inheritance. It should also be added that according to Greek law all children have equal rights to their parents' property. The sons acquire their share mainly through the system of inheritance, whereas the daughters acquire it sooner by getting their dowry.

The Social Rules

> So, all these parents, all these families, all these widows are under the obligation of marrying off all these daughters—five, six, seven of them: and to provide them all with a dowry. . . .And what a dowry according to the customs of the islands: a house at Cotronia, a vineyard at Ammoudia, an olive grove at Lechouni and a field at Stroflia! But recently, in the

> middle of the century, another disease has started to spread. The "counting." Each [parent] was obliged to give also dowry in cash. Two thousand, thousand, five hundred, whatever. Otherwise he had better keep his daughters and admire them. He had better place them on the shelf, lock them up in the wardrobe, send them to the museum.[3]

This is how the well-known Greek novelist Papadiamantis described the social pressure for dowry provision which prevailed in Greece in the 1900s. Two-thirds of a century later these comments have lost nothing of their pertinence. For even today, the penalty that many a poor girl pays for not having a dowry is to remain unmarried, that is, to remain "an old maid" (*a gerontokori),* something which is still considered by the majority of Greeks as one of the worse fates that can befall a woman.

In contemporary Greece two tendencies coexist: on the one hand the tendency to judge a woman's worth as a bride primarily on the basis of the size of her dowry, and on the other, the tendency to judge her primarily on the basis of her educational achievements and, more generally, her whole personality. The first, "traditional" tendency is still more common than the second, more "progressive" one, which has started only recently to gain ground, especially among the better educated and more "Europeanized" Greek families; their attitude is reflected in the motto one hears especially among students, that "A woman's dowry is her education."[4]

The majority of those Greeks, however, who belong to the farmer class, or the working class, or the lower-middle class, continue to regulate the property relations between parents and daughters and between husband and wife on the basis of the rules which emanate from the institution of the dowry. From a purely rational point of view this seems indeed extraordinary, for in most cases their economic interests would be better served if instead of clinging to the tradition of the dowry they broke away, as has happened, for example, in France. Once the parties concerned were in agreement, they could either ignore altogether any legal arrangement to settle the property relations between husband and wife (in this case the couple would decide how each partner should contribute to the household expenses) or choose the legal alternative to the dowry arrangement that the Greek Civil Code provides, the "common pooling of resources" (i.e., *koinoktimosini;* see article 1402 of the Greek Civil Code).

The fact that the institution of the dowry continues to regulate, to a great extent, the property relations between Greek men and women cannot then be explained in terms of the power of its legal norms; the explanation must lie in the power of its social norms which render this institution a highly valued good that each family must at all costs offer to the daughter, and each woman to her husband. Otherwise, the status of the family and of the woman, as well as her chances of marrying or of marrying well, becomes endangered.

Innumerable instances point to the fact that today the dowry is still a powerful status symbol. For example, in Megara, a provincial town near Athens where I did some research a few years ago, the inhabitants are given the opportunity of assessing a girl's trousseau and dowry during the three days preceding the wedding and on the wedding day itself. "It is then that the linen (named the *youko)*, the furniture and the cutlery are exhibited in her [the girl's] house and that neighbors and friends are invited to throw flowers and rice on them [the trousseau items]. One of the aspirations of the Megarian girl is to have a *youko* so voluminous that its pile reaches the ceiling."[5] The origins of this custom may be traced to a time in the past when the society had few status symbols, as was the case with Greek society under the Turkish occupation; thus, the size of the dowry became an important criterion of status and power. Indeed the roots of the modern phenomenon reach far back into the past, whence they draw their strength and their persistence.

The elements which usually compose a dowry—besides the necessary minimum of the trousseau, the household goods, and the furniture—are agricultural property (land, animals, olive trees, etc.), money (usually in gold sovereigns; one gold sovereign equals approximately ten dollars), and residential property (a house or an apartment). Any one of these three elements or a combination of all of them may compose a dowry.[6] Under the existing social pressure for the woman to get as large a dowry as possible, a considerable number of Greek families are faced with an economic problem, which becomes more acute the more daughters they have. Discussions and decisions relating to the question of how to meet the often excessive demands for a large dowry on the part of the daughter's future husband form an inextricable part of the life experience of many a Greek family, and obsessive thoughts on the necessity of acquiring a dowry at all costs still embitter the lives of the Greek young women who come from propertyless families.

The Legal and the Social Reality

On the purely formal, legal level the institution of the dowry has been conceived of as economic assistance by the parents to their daughter and their daughter's family of marriage, the underlying assumption being, of course, that the young woman is not by herself capable of contributing to the expenses of family life (i.e., she cannot share with her husband the role of breadwinner) and that she is not able to look after her own property (hence the husband is to be responsible for its management).

Provided that these assumptions are rooted in reality, as they were in ancient Greece and even in Greek society at the turn of the century, the institution of the dowry has a real and useful purpose: to protect and strengthen the basically weak position of the woman. Once, however, the woman is no more in need of such protection, as is the case today in the most technologically advanced societies and as is becoming increasingly the case in Greece, the institution of the dowry ceases to fulfill any socially useful function. Moreover, in case, for a number of reasons, a woman's chances of marriage come to depend on her ability to provide herself with a dowry, the institution of the dowry defeats its own original purpose, for instead of strengthening the position of the woman, it weakens it considerably, especially in the lower ranks of the socioeconomic hierarchy, which means for the majority of women. This "lag" between the legal conception of the institution of the dowry and the social situation which it generates in practice is encountered undoubtedly in contemporary Greece.

THE INSTITUTION OF THE DOWRY AND ITS MAIN EFFECTS

In discussing the effects of the institution of the dowry under two separate headings, the economic and the social, I am of course aware that this distinction is somewhat artificial, since the economic effects are in the last analysis also social. For purely classificatory purposes, however, this distinction seems useful.

Some Economic Effects

The existence of the institution of the dowry creates strong incentives, especially among the poorer Greek families, to save money over a long period of time, to emigrate, and to work.

Saving. Saving money for the daughter's dowry starts quite often, together with the preparation of her trousseau, at the time of her birth. According to Sanders the process of saving for the dowry starts when the girl is ten years of age and often represents the savings of two generations.[7]

A number of Greek economists have criticized, for obvious reasons, the tendency of Greeks to invest their savings in residential property rather than in industry. There is no doubt that the institution of the dowry, which places demands upon even the poorer families to provide their daughter with a house (be it only a one-room dwelling), is up to a point responsible for this trend.

Emigration. One of the basic reasons why a number of Greek fathers and brothers emigrate from Greece is to get higher wages in order to be able to help the younger females in the family back home with formation of their dowries.

A study conducted a few years ago at the Social Sciences Center of Athens[8] among the families of Greeks who had emigrated to Germany, Belgium, etc., concluded that the great majority of single girls who had emigrated had left Greece in order to earn more and to be able to build up a dowry. It must be added, however, that when Greek young women emigrate, they are in search of not only higher wages but also a non-dowry-oriented society, such as the Australian or the German one, where they may get married to someone who does not demand a dowry.

Female work. In Greece, the wish to form a dowry is very often the decisive factor in a young girl's decision to work. In case the family (that is, the parents or the brothers) is unable to meet the obligation of providing their daughter with a dowry, this burden is shifted automatically onto the girl's shoulders, who now has to work in order to provide herself with a dowry. What in fact happens is that the girl substitutes her earnings for her share in the family property, which she is in no position to get, since there is no such property. This situation could be described as a parody of the institution of the dowry, which actually presupposes the existence of family property. But the influence of this institution has been so far-reaching in this country that it has affected even the propertyless classes. Furthermore, it should be kept in mind that "self-endowment" has a long history in this country.

In Megara, the hope of acquiring a dowry and thus contracting a "successful" marriage proved stronger than all other considerations and provided a powerful incentive for the young women to go to work in the newly built textile factory of Piraiki-Patraiki, and for their mothers to allow them to work there, in spite of the other inhabitants' reactions against the "immorality" of factory work.[9]

It is of interest to note that, ironically enough, it is the existence of a traditional institution—that of the dowry—which encourages female emancipation, for it is very often in order to meet the demands made by tradition that Greek women have to follow a nontraditional way of living, that is, to work outside their own homes either in this country or abroad. At the same time, however, the very fact that such emancipation is used to reinforce traditional norms—i.e., the wages earned are used to form a dowry—leads to a more rapid acceptance of social change than would have been the case in the opposite instance.[10]

Some Social Effects

The institution of the dowry has an impact also on intra- and interfamilial relations, on the age at which young people marry in Greece, as well as on the mechanism of social mobility through marriage.

Intra- and interfamilial relations and the institution of the dowry. Relations first within a girl's family of origin (between, that is, herself, her parents, and her brothers) and later within her family of marriage (between, that is, herself, her husband, and her in-laws) are affected in various ways and in varying degrees by the institution of the dowry.

Campbell, in his thorough study of the inhabitants of a shepherd community of continental Greece, the Sarakatsani, mentions that he encountered among them "women who harbour resentment against their fathers, because, as they allege, they were given to indifferent husbands in order to avoid the payment of a substantial dowry."[11] It is reasonable to assume that such family conflict is not confined only to the Sarakatsani for a number of Greek parents very probably adopt the "lowering of the standard" solution in order to marry off a daughter in case they are either unwilling or unable to give her a sufficiently large dowry; in this case, she will have to restrict her expectations and marry someone who is her inferior in a number of ways and whose demands, for this very reason, are humble.

In a society like that of modern Greece, where, in the countryside, parents are mainly responsible for arranging the marriages of their children and where the kind of marriage a girl makes depends to a large extent on the size of her dowry, which in turn depends on her parents' wealth and goodwill, the daughter may easily come to blame them for her unsuccessful marriage or for her not marrying at all.

In case the parents are unable to shoulder all by themselves the burden of providing their daughter with a dowry, they transfer part of this onto their sons, who, though not legally obliged to help their sister with her dowry, have definitely, however, a moral responsibility in this regard. To those familiar with the history of the institution of the dowry in Greece, it is well known that the brother's responsibility toward his sister's marriage has a very long tradition in this country. Campbell found that among the Sarakatsani the brothers do not claim their legal share in the family property unless all their sisters have gotten married.[12] There are times when the brother gives over to his sister part of what he is legally entitled to inherit from his parents, in order to enable her to marry. This is also mentioned by Friedl in her well-known study of a Boeotian village, Vasilika, where, in case the prospective husband made excessive demands, the girl's brother would add from his own inheritance to her dowry, so that the marriage arrangements would not have to be broken off. According to Friedl, it is in the brother's interest that his sister marry well, because in this way the prestige of the whole family increases, and as a result he is now able in his turn to marry a girl with a substantial dowry.[13]

Naturally, brotherly sacrifice, which leads to closer brother-sister relations, is not always the case. There must be brothers who refuse to help their sister with her dowry, thus giving rise to feelings of resentment against them not only on the part of their sister but very probably also on that of their parents. In conclusion, it is suggested that in case parents and brothers do not offer the girl the dowry she expects or feels she is entitled to get, conflict occurs and intrafamilial relations suffer accordingly.

Relations within the girl's family of marriage are affected by whether she had brought with her a dowry, and if she has, by its size. A woman who brings with her no dower property, which represents additional land and cash for her husband to control and additional property to transmit one day to her children, is from the very start of her marriage at a disadvantage vis-à-vis not only her husband but also her in-laws, becoming a ready target for their criticism and even their contempt; her independence and authority within her own family is thus undermined. By working and contributing through her earnings to the family expenses, she might be able to raise her position, but only somewhat, since from the very start she failed to live up to the expectations long-sanctified by law and custom in regard to the Greek woman.

On the other hand, when her dowry is equal to or even smaller than her husband's property, by the very fact that she has conformed to the expected pattern and has some economic independence, her authority within her home is enhanced. When, however, her dowry markedly exceeds her husband's property, her economic superiority renders her position very powerful indeed, and in this case the authority of her husband might become endangered.[14] As for the usual friction between parents-in-law and daughter-in-law, this is probably mitigated by, as Friedl aptly points out, "the independent dignity a girl acquires by having brought her husband a dowry and by the pride her husband's family takes in their own skill at having helped arrange a good marriage for their son."[15]

The institution of the dowry and the age at marriage. The effect of the institution of the dowry upon the age at which young people marry varies, as logic and a few research findings suggest, according to social class. Among the very poor and the very rich, the institution of the dowry, for very different reasons, favors early marriage: The very poor landless families who can provide their daughters with only a small trousseau and dowry have only one way of increasing their daughter's worth in the marriage market and that is by her chastity; they therefore try their best to marry off their daughters as early as possible, so as to avoid the possibility of their "running wild" and thus forfeiting altogether their already slim marriage chances. This pattern has been observed also by Friedl among the poorer strata of Vasilika.[16] At the other extreme of the social ladder, among the rich and the very rich families, the girl, if she so wishes, can get her dowry at a very young age, and the young man, knowing that he will get a substantial dowry, need not wait a number of years before getting married. At this high socioeconomic level the institution of the dowry on the whole favors early marriage.

However, in the middle ranges of the social hierarchy, where the majority of Greek men and women are found, the institution of the dowry is, in all probability, an obstacle to early marriage. The average farmer's family often needs time to accumulate a dowry which will satisfy the prospective groom's demands. Friedl, for example, found that in Vasilika the age of the girls who marry men from the city (that is, men of higher prestige than their own) is usually twenty-five to thirty.[17] In the urban middle classes marriage tends also to be delayed so that young girls are able to finish the university and get a decent job that will help them increase not only their prestige but also their dowry. Moreover, the majority of Greek young men have to work for a number of years before they are able to shoulder even in part the responsibilities of marriage.

These considerations explain, in part, why Greece (together with Ireland, Italy, Spain, Portugal, and Malta, all countries where the institution of the dowry still functions), when compared with the other European countries, stands out by the relatively late age at which men and women tend to marry.[18]

The institution of the dowry and social mobility through marriage. In the most technologically advanced societies of the West, it seems that "homogamy" (marriage between people of equal wealth and prestige) is becoming the general rule, and "hypergamy" (marriage to someone of higher social and economic status than oneself), whether by the man or the woman, is tending to become the exception.[19] In order to state with any degree of certainty what the trend in this respect is in contemporary Greece, we would need much more empirical evidence, both from rural and from urban areas, than is available at present. In the absence of adequate data, the following hypothesis has to be considered as only tentative: *It is suggested that, in contemporary Greece, upward social mobility through marriage, in other words "hypergamy," tends to take place more often than "homogamy" and is encountered especially among men; this, of course, means that "hypogamy" is more common among women.* The following are some arguments to support this view.

Whereas in the European societies of the past the institution of the dowry tended to encourage the tendency of "homogamy,"[20] in Greece this institution had and has dissimilar effects and seems to encourage mainly "hypergamy" (that is, upward social mobility through marriage) among men. This is largely due to the fact that in Greek society men have been able to create a kind of "dowry inflation" by demanding disproportionately large dowries, disproportionate, that is, to their own means; at the same time, the prospective bride's families have played up to these demands by trying to meet them "at any cost," partly out of a strong sense of responsibility toward the girl, partly out of fear of losing the prospective groom, and last, but not least, out of a sense of honor (*philotimo*) which closely associates dowry provision with family prestige. It should be noted that the interplay of these social forces has its roots in the Greek tradition.

In Greece, marriage is still the main means through which a

woman can acquire full status in the society. On the part, then, of the women within a certain age group (and of their families), there is a strong *demand* for a husband, and, of course, preferably for a socially and economicaly successful one. On the part, however, of the young men in the corresponding or slightly older age group, there is not an equally strong demand for a wife. This is so because the Greek culture exerts a much weaker pressure on the man to get married, especially when he is relatively young, and also because the structure of job opportunity and remuneration in Greek society is still such that a young man has to work for a number of years before he is in a position to cover even the essential expenses of a new household. Under such conditions it is only natural that, within the marriage market and within a given age group, men are valued more highly as husbands than women as wives. As a consequence, women (and their families) are obliged, so to speak, to use strong bait in order to lure men into marriage; conversely, men (and their families) can wait for suitable enticement, thus dictating their own terms for marriage. Given the tremendous force and endurance of the social norms which emanate from the institution of the dowry, playing the game on "their own terms" means asking for as large a dowry as possible; in exchange, the man offers the girl the much sought-after status of being a married woman, and in addition whatever other social assets he may possess. For example, many a rural family values highly the prospective husband who lives in the city,[21] and many a lower-middle-class family, the man with a college degree. The price paid for catching such a husband is a dowry which often exceeds not only the girl's legal share in the family property but also the actual earnings and property of the prospective groom.

Thus, in line with Greek tradition, the institution of the dowry becomes, in practice, abused on both sides, leading to economic hypergamy among the men and to economic hypogamy among the women. Since, however, the acquisition of wealth is also a way to social advancement, hypergamy among men is not just economic but also social. It should be noted, however, that by some criteria, such as education, urban status, etc., Greek men tend to be superior to their wives.

Economic and social considerations are not, of course, always the leading criteria in the choice of a marriage partner. A girl's beauty and personal charm are always strong weapons in the husband-seeking game, and love may override all other considerations. Anyone, however, who lives in Greece today and who is in touch with its countryside and its uneducated classes, realizes that the factors discussed in the preceding paragraphs are still more powerful than the forces of personal feeling in the choice of a marriage partner.

DOWRY, AN INSTITUTION AT THE CROSSROADS BETWEEN PERSISTENCE AND DECLINE

Greek society is, of course, not dominated only by those traditional forces we have described at some length in this article. New trends, such as the increasing participation of women in higher education and in the labor force, and the decreasing influence of the family in the arrangement of marriages, are already at work, especially in Athens and the other large cities. Such trends have already started to undermine the institution of the dowry and in time, as they gradually become stronger and more widespread, will lead to its extinction.

In most European societies the advent of the Industrial Revolution marked a turning point in the history of the institution of the dowry. In brief, the basic changes which followed industrialization and which negatively affected this institution were these: the rise in the educational standard of the population, the increasing participation of women in the labor force, the weakening of the role of the family as matchmaker, and the wide acceptance of a new social ethos which placed greater value upon individual achievement than upon inherited wealth and which recognized the woman's right to play other roles in addition to the strictly biological ones of wife and mother. Today, in the technologically advanced societies, a woman's dowry is her education and her work.

Greece has still quite a long way to go in order to reach this level: in Greek society the institution of the dowry still draws its strength from its economic function within the institution of marriage and from its social function as a powerful status symbol. According to the supporters of the institution of the dowry, it also helps to strengthen the position of the Greek woman by increasing her marriage chances and by enhancing her power within her own family. Greeks, however, are becoming increasingly aware that this institution, and the ways in which it has been abused in practice, has the effect much more often of destroying the marriage chances of the woman, restricting her freedom of choice of a marriage partner, and undermining her position inside the home. This destructive social situation created in Greece by the institution of the dowry cannot but gradually undermine the power of its associated social norms and thus render powerless its legal norms, too. Economic, and especially educational, progress will do the rest.

I wish to acknowledge my indebtedness to the Ford Foundation, whose financial assistance enabled me to study in some detail this aspect of Greek social life. To Professor John Peristiany I would like to express my deep gratitude for recommending me for this grant. Finally, my thanks are also due to Mr. James Warner of the United States Educational Foundation in Greece for the unfailing interest he showed during the completion of this small study, and to my friend and colleague Professor Constantina Safilios-Rothschild, who helped toward its publication.

REFERENCES

1. A case in point is that the definition of the term *dowry* is not given in the recently published *Dictionary of the Social Sciences*, eds. J. Gould and W.L. Kolb (London, 1964); the reader is asked to look up instead *bride-price*, a different, even if related, term.

2. The Civil Code of 1946, on the whole, followed the principles of earlier Byzantine-Roman law, according to which the husband and wife were not under any legal obligation to regulate their property relations according to the rules of the institution of the dowry; by mutual agreement each could retain his/her economic independence. [The dowry laws have recently changed with the Socialist government, but the dowry tradition lingers on.—ed.]

3. A. Papadiamantis, *I Fonissa* [The Murderess], in *Collected Works* (Athens, 1954)1:26-27.

4. Jane Lambiri-Dimaki, "Greek Students: An Analysis of Their Demographic, Social, and Cultural Characteristics," 1969 (unpublished manuscript).

5. Ionna Lambiri, *Social Change in a Greek Country Town* (Athens, 1965), 34-35.

6. See also I. Saunders, *Rainbow in the Rock* (Cambridge, Mass., 1952), 163-5.

7. Ibid, 165-6.

8. The center's name is now National Center of Social Research. For more detailed reference to this research, see Ionna Lambiri-Dimaki, "Dowry in Contemporary Greek Society," *Nea Oikonomia*, no. 11/12 (November-December 1966):886.

9. See Lambiri, *Social Change*, 59-60.

10. Ibid., 94-107.

11. See J.K. Campbell, *Honor, Family, and Patronage* (Oxford, 1964), 172.

12. Ibid., 44.

13. See E. Friedl, *Vasilika, A Village in Modern Greece* (New York, 1962), 66.

14. This point is discussed by E. Friedl in her paper, "The Position of Women : Appearance and Reality," *Anthropological Quarterly* 40 (1967):97-108.

15. Friedl, *Vasilika*, 55.

16. Ibid., 69.

17. Friedl, "The Position of Women," 66.

18. See *European Population Conference* (Strassbourg, 1966), 9-10.

19. See W. Goode, *World Revolution and Family Patterns* (Glencoe, Ill., 1963).

20. See M. Radin, "The Dowry," *The Encyclopedia of the Social Sciences* (New York, 1931), and W.J. Thomas and F. Znaniecki, *The Polish Peasant in Europe and America* (New York, 1958), 87-128.

21. In Vasilika, for example, Friedl found that a girl is considered to have contracted a successful marriage if she marries a man of urban origin. (Friedl, *Vasilika*, 65-66).

Index

